Maternal–Fetal Medicine

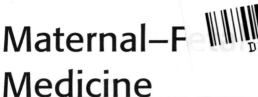

The Queen Elizabeth Hospital
King's Lynn
NHS Trust

CAMBRIDGE UNIVERSITY PRESS
Cambridge, New York, Melbourne, Madrid, Cape Town, Singapore, São Paulo, Delhi

Cambridge University Press
32 Avenue of the Americas, New York, NY 10013-2473, USA

www.cambridge.org
Information on this title: www.cambridge.org/9780521709347

First published 2007

Printed in the United States of America

A catalog record for this publication is available from the British Library.

Library of Congress Cataloging in Publication Data

D'Alton, Mary E.
Maternal-fetal medicine / Mary E. D'Alton, Errol Norwitz, Thomas McElrath.
    p.   cm.
ISBN-13: 978-0-521-70934-7 (pbk.)
ISBN-10: 0-521-70934-2 (pbk.)
1. Fetus – Diseases – Handbooks, manuals, etc.   2. Pregnancy – Complications –
Handbooks, manuals, etc.   3. Prenatal diagnosis – Handbooks, manuals, etc.
I. Norwitz, Errol R.   II. McElrath, Thomas, 1964–   III. Title.
[DNLM: 1. Fetal Diseases–Handbooks.   2. Pregnancy Complications –
Handbooks.   3. Prenatal Diagnosis – Handbooks. WQ 39 D152m 2007]
RG626.D35   2007
618.3'2–dc22   2007016728

ISBN   978-0-521-70934-7 paperback

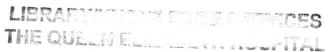

NOTICE

Because of the dynamic nature of medical practice and drug selection and dosage, users are advised that decisions regarding drug therapy must be based on the independent judgment of the clinician, changing information about a drug (e.g., as reflected in the literature and manufacturer's most current product information), and changing medical practices.

While great care has been taken to ensure the accuracy of the information presented, users are advised that the authors, editors, contributors, and publisher make no warranty, express or implied, with respect to, and are not responsible for, the currency, completeness, or accuracy of the information contained in this publication, nor for any errors, omissions, or the application of this information, nor for any consequences arising therefrom. Users are encouraged to confirm the information contained herein with other sources deemed authoritative. Ultimately, it is the responsibility of the treating physician, relying on experience and knowledge of the patient, to determine dosages and the best treatment for the patient. Therefore, the author(s), editors, contributors, and the publisher make no warranty, express or implied, and shall have no liability to any person or entity with regard to claims, loss, or damage caused, or alleged to be caused, directly or indirectly, by the use of information contained in this publication.

Further, the author(s), editors, contributors, and the publisher are not responsible for misuse of any of the information provided in this publication, for negligence by the user, or for any typographical errors.

Contents

Preface   *page* ix

Acute Asthma Exacerbation 1

Acute Cystitis 3

Amniotic Fluid Embolism 5

Antenatal Fetal Testing 7

Antiphospholipid Antibody Syndrome 9

Appendicitis 12

Asthma 14

Asymptomatic Bacteriuria 16

Bacterial Vaginosis 18

Bell's Palsy 20

Breech Presentation 22

Cancer In Pregnancy 24

Cervical Cerclage 26

Cesarean Delivery 29

Chlamydia Trachomatis 31

Chorioamnionitis 33

Chronic Hypertension 35

Cord Prolapse 38

Corticosteroid Therapy 40

Cytomegalovirus 42

Deep Vein Thrombosis 44

Diabetic Ketoacidosis (DKA) 47

Eclampsia 49

Endomyometritis 52

Episiotomy 54

Fetal Bradyarrhythmia 57

Fetal Laboratory Values 59

Fetal Tachyarrhythmia 60

Gestational Diabetes 62

Gonorrhea 65

Group B Streptococcus 67

Headache 69

Hepatitis B 71

Hepatitis C 75

Herpes Simplex Virus 76

Human Immunodeficiency Virus (HIV) 78

Hydrops Fetalis 81

Hyperemesis Gravidarum (HEG) 83

Hyperthyroidism 85

Hypothyroidism 88

Idiopathic Thrombocytopenic Purpura (ITP) 90

Induction of Labor 92

Intrapartum Fetal Testing 95

Intrauterine Fetal Demise 96

Intrauterine Growth Restriction (IUGR) 99

Isoimmunization 101

Listeria 104

Lyme Disease 106

Macrosomia 109

Mastitis 111

Maternal Anemia 113

Maternal Cardiac Disease 116

Maternal Laboratory Values........................118

Multiple Pregnancy................................123

Myasthenia Gravis 126

Obstetric Ultrasound..............................128

Oligohydramnios 130

Operative Vaginal Delivery 133

Paraplegia.......................................135

Parvovirus B19 137

Placenta Accreta 139

Placenta Previa 141

Placental Abruption 144

Pneumonia.......................................146

Polyhydramnios 148

Postpartum Depression............................151

Postpartum Hemorrhage...........................153

Postpartum Psychosis.............................155

Postterm (Prolonged) Pregnancy 157

Preeclampsia 159

Pregestational Diabetes...........................162

Pregnancy-induced Hypertension 165

Prenatal Diagnosis 167

Preterm Labor....................................169

Preterm Prom....................................172

Puerperal Hysterectomy 174

Pulmonary Edema 176

Pulmonary Embolism.............................178

Pyelonephritis 180

Renal Disease 182

Retained Placenta.................................185

Rubella 186

Seizure Disorder 189

Shoulder Dystocia 191

Sickle Cell Hemoglobinopathy 193

Sterilization 196

Syphilis 198

Systemic Lupus Erythematosus (SLE) 200

Term Premature Rupture of Membranes (PROM) 203

Thyroid Storm 205

Toxoplasmosis 207

Trichomoniasis 210

Tuberculosis 212

Vaginal Birth After Cesarean (VBAC) 214

Varicella Zoster 215

Vasa Previa 218

Von Willebrand Disease 220

Preface

Obstetrics is a broad-based specialty requiring expertise in a number of different disciplines, including internal medicine, general surgery, psychiatry, and family medicine. The authors have designed this text to give the reader a succinct yet comprehensive overview of obstetrics using a user-friendly format that is easy to navigate. The text covers topics related to maternal and fetal medicine (such as maternal cardiac and endocrine disorders, infections in pregnancy, and obstetric ultrasound and prenatal diagnosis) as well as clinical questions that will challenge providers both in the outpatient setting (multiple pregnancy, placenta previa, gestational diabetes) and on labor and delivery (such as induction of labor, intrapartum fetal testing, and cesarean delivery to name just a few). Special attention has been paid to incorporating an evidence-based approach to obstetric management, and a number of chapters have been included to assist in the management of obstetric emergencies such as shoulder dystocia, eclampsia, and postpartum hemorrhage. It is the sincere hope of the authors that this text will provide the requisite depth and breadth of knowledge needed to diagnose and manage clinical problems that face obstetric care providers on a daily basis both in the clinic and on labor and delivery.

Mary E. D'Alton, Errol R. Norwitz, and Thomas F. McElrath

ACUTE ASTHMA EXACERBATION

BAKGROUND
- 4% of adult population has asthma
- In general, sx often worsen during 28–36 wk of pregnancy; acute exacerbations rare in last 4 wk or in labor

DIAGNOSIS

History
- Sx include cough, dyspnea, wheezing; fever, chills, malaise less common
- Ask about prior attacks, current Rx, baseline peak expiratory flow rate (PEFR), precipitating events (upper respiratory tract infection, allergen exposure)

Physical examination
- Check temp, pulse oximetry (note: pulse oximetry does *not* assess pt's ability to clear CO_2)
- Examine for cyanosis, hyperinflation, use of accessory muscles, pulsus paradoxus

Diagnostic tests
- *Laboratory tests:* ABG, CBC
- *Specific diagnostic tests:* decrease in PEFR, FEV1
- *Imaging tests:* AP/lateral CXR
- *Screening tests:* daily PEFR

DIFFERENTIAL DIAGNOSIS
- Pulmonary edema
- Pulmonary embolism
- Bronchitis
- Pneumonia

COMPLICATIONS
- *Maternal complications:* respiratory failure, preterm birth

- *Fetal complications:* prematurity, low birthweight, increased perinatal mortality (esp. w/ severe disease)

PROGNOSIS
- Pregnancy represents a state of compensated respiratory alkalosis; maternal PCO_2 >=35 mmHg in room air suggests impending respiratory failure

MANAGEMENT

General measures
- O_2 supplementation to maintain O_2 saturation >=95%, PO_2 >=70%
- Continuous pulse oximetry to follow oxygenation
- Adequate hydration
- Serial ABGs

Specific treatment
- Inhaled beta-2-agonist (bronchodilator) Rx q 20–30 min × 3 doses
- If initial response adequate (ie, increase in PEFR to >=70% predicted or baseline, if known), continue bronchodilator Rx & follow as outpatient
- If response inadequate, continue Rx for 2–3 h; consider admission for measured PEFR <70% predicted
- Consider IV corticosteroid Rx for PEFR 40–70% baseline (or predicted) after 2–3 h
- Stress-dose steroids (IV hydrocortisone 80 mg q8h) in labor if history of steroid Rx in last 6 mo

Contraindications
- Cardiogenic disease relative contraindication to beta-agonist Rx

Side effects & complications of treatment
- Maternal adrenal suppression (can be avoided w/ stress-dose steroids in labor)

Follow-up care
- Regular outpatient visits
- Referral to pulmonologist

SUBSEQUENT MANAGEMENT
- Severity & frequency of acute exacerbations similar in subsequent pregnancies

---

ACUTE CYSTITIS

BACKGROUND
- Most common medical complaint of pregnancy
- Incidence: 1–4% of all pregnancies
- Organisms: *Escherichia coli* (90%), *Staphylococcus saprophyticus* (4–7%)

DIAGNOSIS

History
- Sx may include frequency, dysuria, urgency, suprapubic pain
- *Risk factors:* diabetes, urinary tract anomaly, prior urinary tract infection/pyelonephritis in index pregnancy, sickle cell trait/disease

Physical examination
- Suprapubic tenderness
- Flank pain, costovertebral angle tenderness, fever, systemic complaints usually absent

Diagnostic tests
- Urine dip can be positive for nitrates, leukocyte esterase
- Definitive Dx made by urinalysis (>=100,000 colony-forming units/mL of single pathogenic organism in midstream clean-catch urine specimen)
- Imaging studies not indicated
- Check CBC if patient febrile

DIFFERENTIAL DIAGNOSIS
- Mycotic/bacterial vaginosis w/ contamination of urine specimen
- Asymptomatic bacteriuria
- Pyelonephritis

COMPLICATIONS
- *Maternal complications:* progression to pyelonephritis, urosepsis, ARDS, preterm labor
- *Fetal complications:* preterm birth, low birthweight

PROGNOSIS
- Full resolution can be expected w/ adequate Rx; increased risk of pyelonephritis/urosepsis if Rx inadequate
- Screening/treatment prevents 80% of pyelonephritis in pregnancy

MANAGEMENT
General measures
- Aggressive oral hydration
- Outpatient Rx acceptable in absence of pyelonephritis

Specific treatment
- Antibiotic Rx for 3 d adequate for otherwise healthy women (consider 5-d course for women w/ concurrent chronic disease); single-dose Rx assoc. w/ increased failure rate in pregnancy
- Rx options include trimethoprim/sulfamethoxazole 160/180 mg po bid, nitrofurantoin monohydrate/macrocrystals 100 mg po bid, cephalexin 500 mg po qid
- Adjust Rx according to culture results, if indicated

Prevention
- Periodic screening urinalysis in women at high risk for urinary infections

SUBSEQUENT MANAGEMENT

■ Repeat urine culture in 10 d after completion of Rx ("test of cure")

■ If Rx unsuccessful, consider noncompliance, failed Rx (poor antibiotic selection, antibiotic resistance)

■ Consider suppressive Rx for 6 wk if repeat culture positive w/ same organism.

AMNIOTIC FLUID EMBOLISM

BACKGROUND

■ Rare, unpredictable, catastrophic obstetric event

■ 10% of maternal mortality in U.S.

■ *Incidence:* 1/8,000–1/85,000 births

DIAGNOSIS

History

■ Prodromal sx may include sudden chills, sweating, anxiety

■ *Risk factors:* multiparity, advanced maternal age, hypertonic labor, male fetus, intrauterine fetal demise, oxytocin, amniotomy, abruption, intrauterine pressure catheter, chorioamnionitis, cesarean, preeclampsia, intrauterine saline injection (abortion)

Physical examination

■ *Clinical:* Dx characterized by acute-onset respiratory distress, cyanosis, hypotension, tachycardia, hypoxemia, neurologic manifestations (seizures, coma), hemorrhage in labor/delivery or early puerperium

Diagnostic tests

■ *Laboratory tests:* check CBC, DIC panel

■ *Specific diagnostic tests:* clinical Dx, identification of amniotic fluid (mucin, fetal squames) in pulmonary vasculature at postmortem not pathognomonic

■ *Imaging:* check CXR, V/Q scan (shows decreased perfusion); of little value in acute setting. Transesophageal ultrasound useful in acute assessment of pulmonary embolism in intubated pt.

DIFFERENTIAL DIAGNOSIS
■ Pulmonary embolism
■ Pulmonary edema
■ Venous air embolism (assoc w/ ruptured uterus, placenta previa, persistent atrial septal defect)
■ Aspiration
■ Eclampsia
■ Drug overdose/withdrawal
■ Other causes of DIC

COMPLICATIONS
■ *Maternal complications:* shock, DIC, blood transfusion; very high maternal mortality rate (60–90%), permanent neurologic sequelae (85% of survivors)
■ *Fetal complications:* intrauterine fetal demise, hypoxic ischemic cerebral injury if fetus undelivered

PROGNOSIS
■ Death not inevitable if early Dx, aggressive management, including intubation and possible pulmonary bypass

MANAGEMENT
General measures
■ High index of suspicion, early Dx
■ Monitor vital signs, O_2
■ Anesthesia consult, central hemodynamic monitoring, IV access
■ Immediate delivery regardless of gestational age
■ Rx primarily supportive

Specific treatment

- CPR, Rx hypoxemia (supplemental O_2, mechanical ventilation)
- Control bleeding (correct DIC, uterotonic Rx)
- Correct anemia/coagulopathy w/ aggressive blood product transfusion
- Maintain arterial PO_2 >60 mmHg, O_2 saturation >90%; Rx bronchospasm (terbutaline, aminophylline, ? steroids)
- Maintain SBP >90 mmHg, urine output >25 mL/h; inotropic support (dopamine) as needed

Contraindications

- Regional anesthesia contraindicated in acute setting; general endotracheal anesthesia for cesarean
  - ➤ Airway management crucial and intubation highly likely
  - ➤ Pressor support likely to be acutely needed
  - ➤ May require pulmonary bypass
- Avoid heparin in established DIC

SUBSEQUENT MANAGEMENT

- Recurrence rate not clear, likely low.

ANTENATAL FETAL TESTING

BACKGROUND

- Goal: early identification of fetus at risk for preventable morbidity due to hypoxemia
- Assumptions: (1) hypoxemia leads to permanent injury; (2) tests discriminate between asphyxiated, nonasphyxiated fetuses; (3) early detection can prevent adverse outcome
- At most, 15% of cerebral palsy due to intrapartum hypoxemia

DIAGNOSIS

History

Indications for testing:

1. *Maternal factors:* diabetes, hypertension, hyperthyroidism
2. *Fetal factors:* intrauterine growth restriction, increased fetal activity, oligo/polyhydramnios
3. *Pregnancy-associated:* placental abruption, postterm pregnancy

Physical examination
- Usually unhelpful

Diagnostic tests
1. *Fetal movement charts* ("kick counts"): count all movements in 1 h or count time for 10 kicks; 2–3 times/d; any decreased movement requires further evaluation
2. *Contraction stress test* (CST): measures response of fetal heart rate to contractions (3/10 min required to interpret test); (+) CST defined as decelerations w/ >=50% contractions
3. *Nonstress test* (NST): changes in fetal heart rate pattern w/ time; reflects maturity of fetal autonomic nervous system; absence of reactivity (2 accelerations of 15 bpm × 15 sec in 20 min) depends on gestational age: 50% at 24–28 wk, 15% at 28–32 wk
4. *Biophysical Profile* (BPP): NST + 4 sonographic variables: breathing >=30 sec/30 min, movements >=3/30 min, tone (flexion/extension) >=1/30 min, amniotic fluid volume >=2 cm single vertical pocket

DIFFERENTIAL DIAGNOSIS
Causes of irreversible cerebral injury other than hypoxia:
- Congenital abnormalities
- Intracerebral hemorrhage
- Infection
- Drugs
- Trauma
- Hypotension
- Metabolic (thyroid, hypoglycemia)

COMPLICATIONS
- *Maternal complications:* increased cesarean delivery rate
- *Fetal complications:* iatrogenic prematurity due to false-positive testing

PROGNOSIS
- Negative predictive value (intrauterine fetal demise <1 wk following (−)/reassuring testing) consistent for all tests at 0.3–1.9/1,000 pregnancies
- Positive predictive value varies widely; severely abnormal fetal testing associated w/ adverse outcome in only 25–40% of cases
- Interpret testing in light of gestational age, underlying clinical risk factors, congenital anomalies

MANAGEMENT

General measures
- All antenatal tests probably equally efficacious

Contraindications
- Contraindications to CST: preterm premature rupture of membranes, previa, preterm labor, prior cesarean

SUBSEQUENT MANAGEMENT
- Specific to suspected pathology.

ANTIPHOSPHOLIPID ANTIBODY SYNDROME

BACKGROUND
- Autoimmune disorder characterized by circulating antibodies against membrane phospholipid & one or more specific clinical syndromes
- Incidence depends on population screened (0.5–3% of nonpregnant, 2–4% of pregnant, & 4–5% of women w/ prior pregnancy loss have low-titer anticardiolipin antibody [ACA] IgG;

among women w/ recurrent pregnancy loss, 5–20% have moderate to high titer ACA, & 5–10% are + for lupus anticoagulant [LAC])

DIAGNOSIS

Two elements are required for Dx:

1. **Appropriate clinical setting:**
   - ➤ Recurrent pregnancy loss
   - ➤ Unexplained thrombosis
   - ➤ Autoimmune thrombocytopenia
   - ➤ ? Preeclampsia
   - ➤ ? Intrauterine growth restriction
     AND

2. **A confirmatory serologic test:**
   - ➤ *LAC* is an unidentified antibody causing increases of phospholipid-dependent coagulation tests (aPTT, Russel Viper Venom test) by binding to prothrombin-activator complex; in vivo, LAC causes thrombosis; LAC results reported as present or absent (no titers)
   - ➤ Specific antiphospholipid antibodies measured by ELISA (most commonly ACA) assoc. w/ anticoagulant activity in vitro but procoagulant activity in vivo; ACA IgM alone &/or low-positive IgG may be nonspecific; moderate to high levels of ACA IgG required for Dx
   - ➤ ACA & LAC similar but not identical antibodies; may coexist in vivo (70–80% of women w/ LAC are ACA (+); 10–30% of ACA (+) women have LAC)
   - ➤ False-positive test for syphilis common but not sufficient to make Dx of antiphospholipid antibody syndrome (APS)

DIFFERENTIAL DIAGNOSIS

- ■ SLE (10–30% of women w/ SLE have antiphospholipid antibodies; 60–90% of women w/ APS are ANA (+) but w/ insufficient criteria for Dx of SLE)
- ■ Other causes of thrombocytopenia

COMPLICATIONS

- *Maternal complications:* recurrent pregnancy loss (esp. w/ high-titer ACA), thrombosis (esp. w/ LAC), thrombocytopenia, premature rupture of membranes, preeclampsia, complications of Rx (hemorrhage, osteoporosis, fractures, cataracts, infection, adrenal suppression)
- *Fetal complications:* prematurity, placental abruption, intrauterine growth restriction, stillbirth

PROGNOSIS

- If untreated, risk of pregnancy loss in a woman w/ APS & prior pregnancy loss is 60%, whereas 60–70% of women deliver viable infant if treated

MANAGEMENT

General measures

- Weight of evidence suggests that Rx beneficial for APS & prior pregnancy loss
- Rx options include acetylsalicylic acid (ASA), prednisone, heparin, alone or in combination
- Alternative Rx options (intravenous IgG, azathioprine, plasmapheresis) of unclear benefit

Specific treatment

- Low-dose ASA (60–100 mg daily) + prophylactic heparin Rx of choice; no proven benefit of therapeutic over prophylactic heparin
- Low-dose ASA + prednisone (40–60 mg daily) alternative Rx option
- Heparin & prednisone should not be given together due to additive risk of osteoporosis
- Rx should be initiated early in pregnancy & continued to delivery
- Regular fetal testing (serial ultrasound examinations for fetal growth)
- Consider scheduling delivery at 39–40 wk

SUBSEQUENT MANAGEMENT

Prevention
- Women w/ APS & history of thrombosis should probably be treated for life to prevent a catastrophic thrombotic event

Future pregnancies
- Subsequent pregnancies at risk for spontaneous abortion & other complications
- Circulating levels of autoantibodies do not correlate w/ clinical features.

APPENDICITIS

BACKGROUND
- Most common nonobstetric surgical emergency in pregnancy
- Incidence: 1/2,000 pregnancies
- 1st trimester > 2nd or 3rd trimester
- Incidence not increased compared w/ nonpregnant population but more difficult Dx to make & appendix more likely to perforate in pregnancy

DIAGNOSIS

History
- Sx include anorexia, chills, nausea, vomiting, abdominal pain, malaise
- No known risk factors

Physical examination
- Low- to moderate-grade fever
- 1st & early 2nd trimesters: RLQ pain w/ rebound, guarding
- Late 2nd & 3rd trimesters: pain may be diffuse or localized to RLQ or RUQ w/ rebound, guarding

Diagnostic tests
- Dx requires a high index of clinical suspicion

- Check CBC w/ differential
- Early surgical consultation
- Imaging studies not necessary but commonly recommended; abdominal ultrasound of unclear usefulness in pregnancy; consider abdominal CT if available
    - ➤ Fine-cut imaging improves sensitivity and minimizes fetal exposure
- Definitive Dx relies on pathologic exam of appendix (1/3 of appendices "negative" in pregnancy)

DIFFERENTIAL DIAGNOSIS
- Biliary disease
- Lower lobe pneumonia
- Pyelonephritis
- Pancreatitis
- Ovarian torsion
    - ➤ Rupture or hemorrhage of ovarian cyst
    - ➤ Mesenteric adenitis

COMPLICATIONS
- *Maternal complications:* perforation (25% in pregnancy), sepsis, preterm labor & delivery
- *Fetal complications:* spontaneous abortion (17–21% fetal loss rate in setting of perforation), preterm birth, increased risk of neuro damage to neonates delivered after acute inflammation of appendicitis

PROGNOSIS
- Prognosis good w/ prompt Dx & surgical intervention

MANAGEMENT
General measures
- Hydration, antipyretic Rx as needed
- Optimize pain control

Specific treatment
- Prompt surgical intervention Rx of choice
- Laparoscopic appendectomy acceptable if technically feasible
- Technical considerations: left lateral tilt on OR table if >20 wk; continuous intraoperative fetal monitoring if >24 wk; consider right paramedian skin incision
- Consider intra- & postoperative tocolysis (indomethacin)
- Antibiotics (ampicillin, gentamicin, clindamycin) in perioperative period

Follow-up care
- Routine postsurgical follow-up

SUBSEQUENT MANAGEMENT

Prevention
- No place for prophylactic (elective) appendectomy at cesarean delivery
- Future pregnancies unaffected

ASTHMA

BACKGROUND
- 4% of adult population have asthma
- 33–50% of women have no change in sx in pregnancy; 25–33% improve; 25–33% worsen (severe asthma more likely to worsen)
- Sx often worsen at 28–36 wk; acute exacerbations rare in last 4 wk of pregnancy or in labor

DIAGNOSIS

History
- Sx include cough, dyspnea, wheezing

■ Ask about prior attacks, current Rx, baseline peak expiratory flow rate (PEFR), precipitating events (upper respiratory tract infection, allergen exposure)

Physical examination
■ Check temp, pulse oximetry
■ Examine for cyanosis, clubbing, wheezing

Diagnostic tests
■ *Laboratory tests:* none
■ *Specific diagnostic tests:* check pulmonary tests (FEV1, FVC, FEV1/FVC)
■ *Imaging tests:* not routinely indicated
■ *Screening tests:* daily PEFR

DIFFERENTIAL DIAGNOSIS
■ COPD
■ Bronchitis/pneumonia

COMPLICATIONS
■ *Maternal complications:* acute flare, status asthmaticus, respiratory failure
■ *Fetal complications:* prematurity, low birthweight

PROGNOSIS
■ Increased risk of preterm birth, low birthweight
■ Increase in perinatal mortality (esp. w/ severe disease)

MANAGEMENT

General measures
■ Optimize medical, behavioral management
■ Remove environmental precipitants
■ Monitor PEFR daily

Specific treatment
■ Mild disease (PEFR >=80% expected or baseline, if known, w/ symptoms <=2x/wk), treat w/ inhaled beta-2-agonist during sx

- Moderate disease (60–80% PEFR w/ sx >2x/wk), treat w/ inhaled beta-2-agonist, inhaled steroids
- Severe disease (<60% PEFR w/ frequent/nocturnal sx), treat w/ inhaled beta-2-agonist, inhaled steroids, & consider systemic steroids
- Stress-dose steroids (IV hydrocortisone 80 mg q8h) in labor if history of steroid Rx in past 6 mo
- Monitor fetal growth
- Fentanyl & epidural for pain management in labor (avoid excess meperidine, morphine because of respiratory depression)

Contraindications
- Use of prostaglandins (esp. PGF2-alpha) can worsen symptoms

Side effects & complications of treatment
- Maternal adrenal suppression (may require stress-dose steroids in labor)
- Oral thrush (secondary to steroids)

Follow-up care
- Regular outpatient visits
- Referral to pulmonologist

SUBSEQUENT MANAGEMENT
- Course of asthma exacerbations similar in subsequent pregnancies

---

ASYMPTOMATIC BACTERIURIA

BACKGROUND
- Refers to persistent bacterial colonization of urinary tract in absence of urinary tract sx
- Complicates 5–10% of pregnancies

- Not more common in pregnancy but more likely to be symptomatic & progress to pyelonephritis
- Most common pathogen *Escherichia coli* (65–80%)

DIAGNOSIS

History
- Asymptomatic
- *Risk factors:* diabetes mellitus, UTI/pyelonephritis in index pregnancy, sickle cell trait/disease

Physical examination
- Benign (no suprapubic or costovertebral angle tenderness)

Diagnostic tests
- Urine dip can be positive for nitrates, leukocyte esterase
- Definitive Dx made by urinalysis (>=100,000 colony-forming units/mL of single pathogenic organism in midstream clean-catch urine specimen)
- Imaging studies not indicated

DIFFERENTIAL DIAGNOSIS
- Contamination w/ lower genital tract organisms
- Acute cystitis (if symptomatic)
- Pyelonephritis

COMPLICATIONS
- *Maternal complications:* progresses to symptomatic urinary infection (cystitis, pyelonephritis), urosepsis, ARDS, preterm labor, transient renal dysfunction, anemia
- *Fetal complications:* sepsis (rare), low birthweight, preterm birth

PROGNOSIS
- Progression to pyelonephritis in 13–65% of women if untreated; in 2.9% of women if treated

- Screening/treatment prevents 80% of pyelonephritis in pregnancy

MANAGEMENT

General measures
- Aggressive oral hydration

Specific treatment
- Antibiotic Rx for 7–10 d because of high recurrence rate
- Rx options include trimethoprim/sulfamethoxazole 160/180 mg po bid, nitrofurantoin 100 mg po bid, cephalexin 500 mg po qid
- Adjust Rx according to culture results, if indicated

Prevention
- Consider screening w/ urine dip/culture at first antenatal visit
- Consider repeat urinalysis at 16–18 wk; q mo for women w/ sickle cell trait/disease

SUBSEQUENT MANAGEMENT
- Repeat urine culture in 10 d after completion of Rx ("test of cure")
- If Rx unsuccessful, consider noncompliance, failed Rx (poor antibiotic selection, antibiotic resistance)
- Consider suppressive Rx for 6 wk if recurrence w/ same organism after Rx or progression to symptomatic infection

---

BACTERIAL VAGINOSIS

BACKGROUND
- Results from vaginal overgrowth of several organisms, incl. *Bacteroides, Peptostreptococcus, Gardnerella vaginalis, Mycoplasma hominis, Enterobacteriaceae*
- Incidence: 10–25% in low-risk obstetric population; 65% in specialty sexually transmitted disease clinics

- Symptomatic women at increased risk for preterm delivery but insufficient evidence that Rx significantly decreases risk

DIAGNOSIS

History

- 50% of patients asymptomatic
- Sx may include scant or thin malodorous discharge, vaginal pain or burning; sx may increase after menses or intercourse (due to change in vaginal pH)
- Vulvar pruritus usually not present

Physical examination

- Dx made by wet smear w/ >=2 of following 4 criteria:
- Wet mount positive for clue cells
- Decrease in abundance of lactobacilli
- Positive "whiff test" (fishy odor) on mixture w/ potassium hydroxide
- Vaginal pH >4.5

Diagnostic tests

- *Laboratory tests:* check wet prep, vaginal pH
- *Specific diagnostic tests:* none; bacterial vaginosis clinical Dx based on exam, wet prep, & high index of clinical suspicion
- *Imaging tests:* none indicated

DIFFERENTIAL DIAGNOSIS

- Trichomoniasis
- Vaginal candidiasis
- Gonorrhea
- Cervicitis

COMPLICATIONS

- *Maternal complications:* increased risk of preterm delivery in symptomatic women (& possibly in asymptomatic women at high risk for preterm birth)
- *Fetal complications:* none (not assoc. w/ chorioamnionitis)

PROGNOSIS

- >90% cure if compliant w/ Rx

MANAGEMENT

General measures

- Despite association between bacterial vaginosis & preterm birth, Rx has not been shown to effective; therefore routine screening of asymptomatic women not recommended

Specific treatment

- 1st trimester: clindamycin 2% cream vaginally qhs × 7 d
- 2nd/3rd trimesters: metronidazole (Flagyl) 500mg po bid × 7 d

Contraindications

- Allergy or sensitivity to therapeutic agents

Side effects & complications of treatment

- Antabuse-like effect if alcohol consumed while on metronidazole
- Increased diarrhea w/ oral clindamycin

Follow-up care

- Follow-up test of cure required

SUBSEQUENT MANAGEMENT

- Evaluate risk for other sexually transmitted diseases

BELL'S PALSY

BACKGROUND

- Acute, isolated, lower motor neuron facial palsy of unknown cause likely due to inflammation, edema of facial nerve as it exits skull via stylomastoid foramen, leading to axonal degeneration & denervation of facial muscles
- Occurs at any age, males = females

- *Incidence:* 45/100,000 in pregnancy (vs. 17–25/100,000 in nonpregnant reproductive-age women)
- Increases in 2nd/3rd trimester, puerperium

DIAGNOSIS

History
- Ask about onset (usually acute onset w/ maximal weakness <48 h)
- Associated sx: hyperacusis, pain, epiphora (tearing), disturbance of taste
- *Risk factors:* diabetes, pregnancy, hypertension (not preeclampsia), dental anesthesia, ? herpes simplex virus

Physical examination
- Clinical Dx; confirm isolated lower (not upper) motor neuron palsy
- Exclude other neurologic features

Diagnostic tests
- *Laboratory tests:* none
- *Specific diagnostic tests:* may include EMG studies, nerve biopsy, but not routinely indicated
- *Imaging tests:* not indicated

DIFFERENTIAL DIAGNOSIS
- Upper motor neuron facial palsy (usually pontine lesion)
- Facial hemispasm
- Multiple sclerosis
- Simultaneous bilateral facial weakness may suggest meningitis, HIV, sarcoidosis, Lyme disease

COMPLICATIONS
- *Maternal complications:* permanent facial palsy (10%), eye infections
- *Fetal complications:* unaffected

PROGNOSIS
- Typically resolves over days to weeks; 10% have severe & permanent disfigurement
- Poor prognostic features include complete palsy, pain, advanced age, loss of taste, no resolution in 4 wk
- Pregnancy does not alter natural course of paralysis

MANAGEMENT

General measures
- Rx aimed at decreasing inflammation around facial nerve
- Steroids may affect outcome but evidence suggests they do not hasten resolution or improve prognosis
- Neurology consult, if indicated

Specific treatment
- Consider short course of high-dose prednisone (80 mg/d tapered over 10 d)
- Surgery to decompress facial nerve has not shown any benefit

SUBSEQUENT MANAGEMENT
- Recurrent Bell's palsy common

BREECH PRESENTATION

BACKGROUND
- Refers to fetus presenting buttocks first
- *Types:* frank (70%), complete (10%), footling/incomplete (20%)
- *Incidence:* 3–4% at term

DIAGNOSIS

History
- Confirm gestational age
- Fetal movements unhelpful in Dx

■ *Risk factors:* prematurity (28% at 28 wk, 15% at 30 wk), uterine anomalies, polyhydramnios, prior breech, multiple pregnancy, previa, fetal anomalies (anencephaly, goiter, hydrocephaly)

Physical examination

■ Check presentation by Leopold maneuvers, bimanual exam
■ Check position of breech by bimanual exam (defined relative to sacrum)

Diagnostic tests

■ *Imaging tests:* ultrasound to confirm Dx; check gestational age, associated factors (multiple pregnancy, uterine/fetal anomalies, polyhydramnios)

DIFFERENTIAL DIAGNOSIS

■ Transverse, oblique lie
■ Variable/unstable lie

COMPLICATIONS

■ *Maternal complications:* preterm delivery, pelvic trauma
■ *Fetal complications:* cord prolapse, increased risk of birth injury (incl. entrapment of aftercoming head), 2x increased congenital anomaly

PROGNOSIS

■ Term breech presentation increases adverse perinatal outcome, independent of route of delivery

MANAGEMENT

General measures

■ Preterm singleton breech should be delivered by cesarean
■ Vaginal breech delivery of 2nd twin safe (esp. >32 wk, estimated fetal weight >1,500 g & <3,500 g, concordant) Several authors suggest that long-term neuro damage is more

common among breech-delivered second twins. Consider abdominal delivery.

Specific treatment

- Term breech should be delivered abdominally (increased risk of head entrapment, asphyxia, cord prolapse, birth trauma w/ vaginal breech delivery)
- Consider external cephalic version (ECV) >36 wk; 50–70% success rate (higher if frank, nonengaged, normal fluid, multipara, nonobese, lateral fetal spine, use of epidural/uterine relaxant)
- Vaginal delivery of term singleton breech may be considered if frank breech, estimated fetal weight 2,500–4,000 g, head not hyperextended, adequate pelvimetry, experienced operator, capacity for emergent cesarean)

Side effects & complications of treatment

- Cord accident, abruption, fetal distress, premature rupture of membranes, isoimmunization (RhoGAM, if indicated)

Contraindications

- *Absolute:* uterine anomalies, previa, bleeding, premature rupture of membranes, twins, nonreassuring fetal testing
- *Relative:* prior cesarean, intrauterine growth restriction, labor, oligohydramnios

SUBSEQUENT MANAGEMENT

- Cesarean for breech has implications for future pregnancies (risk of uterine rupture, abnormal placentation)

CANCER IN PREGNANCY

BACKGROUND

- Counseling must balance risk to fetus of Rx & prematurity against the risk to mother of delaying Rx

- Most common malignancies of young: breast, lymphoma, leukemia, melanoma, colon, ovary, thyroid

DIAGNOSIS

History
- Sx specific to malignancy

Physical examination
- Note possible metastases (including lymph nodes)

Diagnostic tests
- *Laboratory tests:* check baseline hepatic, renal function
- *Specific diagnostic tests:* if indicated, check tumor marker
- *Imaging tests:* as indicated

DIFFERENTIAL DIAGNOSIS
- Specific for malignancy under Rx

COMPLICATIONS
- *Maternal complications:* depend on specific malignancy
- *Fetal complications:* iatrogenic prematurity, metastases to fetus (rare, only w/ melanoma)

PROGNOSIS
- Pregnancy does not appear to worsen outcome or disease progression

MANAGEMENT

General measures
- Multidisciplinary approach
- If a realistic chance of cure or significant prolongation of survival of mother, pregnancy should not delay Rx; if cure unrealistic, Rx should minimize effects to fetus

Specific treatment
- Consider pregnancy termination if excessive exposure to chemotherapeutic agents or radiation anticipated in early pregnancy

Side effects & complications of treatment

- Effects of *chemotherapy* depend on drug, dose/duration of Rx, gestational age: (1) in 1st trimester, teratogenicity ~6% w/ single agent, 90–100% w/ folate antagonists; (2) in 2nd/3rd trimesters, no evidence of structural injury or developmental delay, but data limited
- Effects of *radiation* depend on type, dose/duration, gestational age: (1) in 1st trimester, 0.5–1 Gy (5–10 rad) may cause abortion; (2) at 3–10 wk, >50% of fetuses exposed to >2.5 Gy have mental retardation, microcephaly, retinal degeneration, cataracts, skeletal abnormalities, intrauterine growth restriction; (3) at 12–20 wk, may cause intrauterine growth restriction, microcephaly, mental retardation; (4) >20 wk, no anomalies
- Surgery least likely to affect fetus; oophorectomy <9–12 wk may require progesterone supplementation; cervical surgery in pregnancy may increase risk of pregnancy loss

SUBSEQUENT MANAGEMENT

- Cancer recurrence not more likely in subsequent pregnancy

CERVICAL CERCLAGE

BACKGROUND

- Cervical insufficiency (CI) refers to inability to support pregnancy to term due to functional defect of cervix
- Incidence: 0.05–1% of pregnancies

DIAGNOSIS

History

- Usually asymptomatic
- May present w/ preterm premature rupture of membranes, watery vaginal discharge, pelvic pressure in midtrimester, prolapse of fetal membranes or products of conception

- *Risk factors:* prior CI, in utero diethylstilbestrol exposure, cervical surgery, or trauma (controversial)

Physical examination
- Confirm painless cervical dilatation in absence of uterine contractions
- Funneling, shortened cervix on ultrasound may suggest Dx

Specific diagnostic tests
- CI a *clinical* Dx in pregnancy (cannot reliably make Dx prior to pregnancy)

DIFFERENTIAL DIAGNOSIS
- Preterm labor
  ➣ Preterm premature rupture of fetal membranes

COMPLICATIONS
- *Maternal complications:* preterm premature rupture of membranes, intra-amniotic infection
- *Fetal complications:* prematurity

PROGNOSIS
- Natural Hx of CI is acute, painless cervical dilatation in midtrimester culminating in preterm PROM, preterm & often pre-viable delivery

MANAGEMENT
General measures
- Transvaginal cerclage Rx of choice for CI
- Elective (prophylactic) cerclage can prevent CI in women at high risk; up to 25 cerclages may be needed to maintain 1 pregnancy
- Prior CI only indication for elective cerclage (cerclage for diethylstilbestrol, short cervix, multiple pregnancy w/o prior pregnancy loss are controversial)

- Emergent (therapeutic) cerclage and cerclage for a shortened cervical length have questionable efficacy in improving perinatal outcome.

Specific treatment
- Shirodkar, McDonald transvaginal cerclage equally efficacious
- Transabdominal cerclage more morbid procedure; should be reserved for cases in which transvaginal cerclage has failed; requires significant expertise & pt counseling
- *Technical considerations:* exclude contraindications prior to placement; check fetal viability before & after procedure; no proven benefit of routine tocolysis or antibiotics for elective cerclage

Contraindications
- *Absolute:* chorioamnionitis, intrauterine fetal demise, lethal fetal anomaly, vaginal bleeding, preterm PROM, >=28 wk
- *Relative:* intrauterine growth restriction, previa, prolapsing membranes, >=24 wk

Side effects and complications
- Increases w/ gestational age & cervical dilatation
- *Short-term (<48 h):* preterm PROM, hemorrhage, pregnancy loss (3–20%)
- *Long-term:* cervical laceration (3–4%), chorioamnionitis (4%), cervical stenosis (1%), puerperal infection (6% vs. 3% w/o cerclage), other (intrauterine fetal demise, placental abruption, thrombophlebitis, abdominal pain)
- If membranes prolapsing, risk of iatrogenic rupture of membranes 40–50%; filling the bladder, Trendelenburg position, therapeutic amniocentesis may help to reduce membranes prior to cerclage placement

Follow-up care
- Frequent visits for cervical checks

- Consider bed rest, "pelvic rest" (no coitus, tampons, douching)
- Remove cerclage electively at 37 wk or w/ uterine contractions (to avoid cervical laceration, uterine rupture)
- Whether or not to remove a cerclage in setting of preterm PROM is unclear; evidence of infection should prompt immediate removal

SUBSEQUENT MANAGEMENT
- CI recurs in 15–30% of subsequent pregnancies
- Elective cerclage should be offered to women w/ Hx of CI in all future pregnancies

CESAREAN DELIVERY

BACKGROUND
- Refers to delivery via abdominal route (laparotomy) requiring incision into uterus (hysterotomy)
- 2nd most common surgery in U.S. (behind circumcision), accounting for 25% of all deliveries

DIAGNOSIS

History
- Ask about prior surgery, allergies, underlying medical conditions
- Written consent

Physical examination
- Check airway (Mallampati classification)

Diagnostic tests
- *Laboratory tests:* check CBC, type & screen
- *Specific diagnostic tests:* none
- *Imaging tests:* not routinely indicated

DIFFERENTIAL DIAGNOSIS

■ Most common reason for primary cesarean is failure to progress in labor; consider inadequate uterine contractions that can be augmented by oxytocin, artificial rupture of membranes

COMPLICATIONS

■ *Maternal complications:* infection, hemorrhage (mean estimated blood loss at cesarean is 1,000 mL), blood transfusion, injury to adjacent organs (bowel, bladder, ureter), need for further surgery (hysterectomy, bowel repair)

■ *Fetal complication:* traumatic injury (rare)

PROGNOSIS

■ Increases risk of bleeding, infection, thromboembolism compared w/ vaginal delivery

MANAGEMENT

General measures

■ Indications for cesarean:
  ➤ Maternal (failure to progress, cephalopelvic disproportion, elective repeat, maternal disease, ? maternal request)
  ➤ Uteroplacental (previa, abruption, prior "classic" cesarean, prior uterine rupture, cord prolapse)
  ➤ Fetal (nonreassuring fetal testing, malpresentation, ? macrosomia, ? fetal anomaly)

Specific treatment

■ Consider amniocentesis for lung maturity prior to elective cesarean <39 wk

■ Regional preferred over general anesthesia (decreases respiratory complications, faster postoperative recovery)

■ *Skin incision* may be Pfannenstiel (low transverse, muscle separating, strong, but limited exposure), midline vertical (best exposure but weak)

- Lower uterine segment transverse *hysterotomy* preferred (decreases blood loss, strong); consider lower segment vertical &/or high vertical ("classic") hysterotomy only if limited access to or poorly developed lower segment, transverse lie, previa, large abnormal fetus (hydrocephalus), extreme prematurity, planned hysterectomy
- Prophylactic antibiotics (2nd-generation cephalosporin) after clamping of cord

Contraindications
- No elective surgery (myomectomy) at cesarean because increases bleeding

SUBSEQUENT MANAGEMENT
- Subsequent pregnancies at risk of uterine rupture

CHLAMYDIA TRACHOMATIS

BACKGROUND
- Cause of most common sexually transmitted disease in U.S.
- Obligate intracellular parasite (cannot generate adenosine triphosphate, therefore dependent on host energy supply)
- Incidence in pregnancy ranges from 2–24%, depending on population (5% average w/in U.S.)

DIAGNOSIS
History
- May be asymptomatic
- Sx include vaginal itching, discharge
- *Risk factors:* unmarried, age <20 y, partner w/ urethritis, other sexually transmitted diseases, late/no prenatal care

Physical examination
- Mucopurulent cervicitis & vaginal discharge
- Red, inflamed ("strawberry") cervix

Diagnostic tests
- *Laboratory tests:* urine culture & analysis for sterile pyuria; check rapid plasma reagin, gonococcal, & HIV tests
- *Specific diagnostic tests:* (1) polymerase chain reaction-based tests sensitive & appropriate for low-incidence populations; (2) antigen detection methods (ELISA, fluorescein-conjugated antibody test) less reliable in low-incidence populations; (3) cytologic staining largely replaced by polymerase chain reaction or antigen-based screening
- *Imaging tests:* not useful

DIFFERENTIAL DIAGNOSIS
- Urinary tract infection
- Gonococcal cervicitis
- HIV infection

COMPLICATIONS
- *Maternal complications:* mucopurulent cervicitis, acute urethral syndrome, rectal & pharyngeal infection, possible increased risk of preterm premature rupture of membranes/preterm labor
- *Fetal complications:* conjunctivitis (most common cause in first month of life), neonatal pneumonia

PROGNOSIS
- 60–70% of neonates exposed at delivery become infected (25–50% develop conjunctivitis; 10–20% develop pneumonia w/in 4 mo of birth)

MANAGEMENT
General measures
- Screen all women in 1st trimester
- Assess risk factors; rescreen high-risk patients in 3rd trimester

Specific treatment
- Topical treatment inadequate

■ Appropriate Rx: amoxicillin, 500 mg po tid × 7 d; erythromycin base, 500 mg po qid × 7 d; azithromycin, 1 g po × 1 (efficacy of last regimen not proved in pregnancy)

Contraindications

■ Known allergies to above agents

Follow-up care

■ Negative test of cure should be obtained 2 wk after Rx

SUBSEQUENT MANAGEMENT

■ Consider rescreening later in pregnancy
■ Consider testing partner

CHORIOAMNIONITIS

BACKGROUND

■ Incidence: 1% of all pregnancies
■ Primarily ascending infection typically following rupture of fetal membranes, although 5% of cases of chorioamnionitis occur in setting of intact membranes; in rare cases (such as *Listeria*), maternal bacteremia can seed amniotic space
■ Most infections polymicrobial (*Escherichia coli, Klebsiella, Bacteroides*, group B beta-hemolytic streptococci, *Fusobacterium, Clostridium, Peptostreptococcus*); mild subclinical infections may be assoc. w/ *Mycoplasma, Ureaplasma, Fusobacterium*

DIAGNOSIS

History

■ Sx incl. chills, abdominal pain, uterine contractions, malaise
■ *Risk factors:* preterm premature rupture of membranes, multiple vaginal exams, bacterial vaginosis

Physical examination

■ Classic clinical features incl. fever, fundal tenderness, maternal &/or fetal tachycardia
■ Malodorous vaginal discharge

Diagnostic tests
- Intra-amniotic infection *clinical* Dx
- Check CBC, blood culture
- Consider amniocentesis: amniotic fluid culture gold standard for Dx; other amniotic fluid features suggestive of infection incl. glucose <=20 mg/dL, leukocytes, bacteria on Gram stain (only 30–50% sensitivity)
- No place for radiologic imaging to confirm Dx

DIFFERENTIAL DIAGNOSIS
- Appendicitis
- Cystitis
- Pyelonephritis
- Mesenteric adenitis

COMPLICATIONS
- *Maternal complications:* sepsis, increase in cesarean delivery rate, postpartum endometritis, preterm labor/delivery, ARDS
- *Fetal complications:* sepsis, preterm birth & sequelae of prematurity, increased risk of cerebral palsy

PROGNOSIS
- Maternal prognosis good w/ prompt Dx & Rx; maternal death rare
- Neonatal mortality/morbidity related primarily to gestational age

MANAGEMENT
General measures
- Inpatient management
- Antipyretic Rx, analgesia as needed

Specific Rx
- Immediate delivery only definitive Rx, ideally w/in 12 h
- Infection not an indication for cesarean delivery

- Initiate broad-spectrum antibiotics: ampicillin 2 g IV q4–6h plus gentamicin 1.5 mg/kg IV q8h; consider adding clindamycin 900 mg IV q8h to cover anaerobes
- Continue antibiotics until 24–48 h afebrile, asymptomatic

Side effects & complications of treatment
- Adverse reaction to specific antibiotic
- Risk of Asherman's syndrome, esp. if infected postpartum

SUBSEQUENT MANAGEMENT
- No follow-up cultures necessary
- Future pregnancies rarely affected

CHRONIC HYPERTENSION

BACKGROUND
- Hypertensive diseases of pregnancy (chronic hypertension, gestational hypertension, preeclampsia) are 2nd most common cause of maternal death in U.S. (behind embolism), accounting for 15% of all maternal deaths/y
- Refers to hypertension prior to pregnancy w/ or w/o treatment; consider Dx in women w/ sustained elevation in BP >=140/90 mmHg prior to 20 wk gestation

DIAGNOSIS
History
- Usually asymptomatic
- May present w/ headache
- *Risk factors:* coexisting maternal disease (chronic renal insufficiency, diabetes, hyperlipidemia, pheochromocytoma), family Hx, advanced maternal age

Physical examination
- Check BP (use appropriate-size BP cuff, pt should be sitting at rest, use disappearance of sounds [5th Korotkoff sound] for diastolic measurement in pregnancy)

- Examine for features of longstanding hypertension (eg, retinal changes)
- Examine for features of underlying coexisting medical conditions

Diagnostic tests
- Remains *clinical* diagnosis based on serial BP measurements
- Check baseline liver function tests, platelet count, proteinuria, renal function in 2nd trimester (given increased risk of superimposed preeclampsia)
- Consider evaluation for cause of chronic hypertension (ultrasound to exclude renal artery stenosis, 24-h urinary VMA or total catecholamines for pheochromocytoma)

DIFFERENTIAL DIAGNOSIS
- Other hypertensive disorders of pregnancy (gestational hypertension, preeclampsia)
- Pheochromocytoma
- Complication of drug therapy (eg, long-term corticosteroid therapy)
- Drug withdrawal, esp. cocaine
- False-positive BP measurement (BP cuff too small, pt not at rest)

COMPLICATIONS
- *Maternal complications:* increased risk of superimposed preeclampsia, placental abruption, stroke, maternal mortality; long-term risk of progression to cardiovascular disease
- *Fetal complications:* uteroplacental insufficiency & intrauterine growth restriction, stillbirth

PROGNOSIS
- Depends on underlying cause, severity of hypertension, gestational age, treatment regimen, & presence of complications (superimposed preeclampsia)

MANAGEMENT

General measures

- Consult w/ pt prior to conception
- In general, continue antihypertensive medications w/ exception of angiotensin-converting enzyme (ACE) inhibitor drugs, which should be discontinued; beta-blocker & calcium channel blocker drugs well tolerated in pregnancy; diuretics generally discouraged in pregnancy

Specific treatment

- Follow BP regularly in pregnancy; evaluate for superimposed preeclampsia if evidence of new-onset proteinuria or significant increase in baseline BP
- Modify treatment regimen as needed (not empirically)
- Regular fetal testing (serial ultrasound examinations for fetal growth; weekly nonstress test, Doppler, amniotic fluid index if evidence of growth restriction)
- Mode & timing of delivery depend on severity of hypertension, condition & gestational age of fetus, condition of mother; in general, delivery should be achieved by 40 wk

Side effects & complications of treatment

- ACE inhibitor (enalapril) use in 1st trimester not assoc. w/ increase in structural anomalies as compared w/ baseline incidence of 1.5–2% but is assoc. w/ functional renal injury (only partially reversed after delivery) & w/ oligohydramnios
- An assoc. described between beta-blockers & oligohydramnios, but controversial

SUBSEQUENT MANAGEMENT

- Pts should follow up w/ primary care provider postpartum
- Complications (eg, superimposed preeclampsia) may recur in a subsequent pregnancy

CORD PROLAPSE

BACKGROUND
- Refers to passage of umbilical cord into vagina following rupture of membranes ahead of presenting part at any gestational age
- Complicates 0.4% of term cephalic pregnancies

DIAGNOSIS

History
- History of premature rupture of membranes
- May present w/ prolapse of cord out of vagina, decreased fetal movement
- Risk factors: malpresentation (0.5% of frank breech, 4–6% complete breech, 5–18% footling breech, 20% transverse lie); amniotomy (artificial rupture of membranes [AROM]); prematurity; small fetus (intrauterine growth restriction or small for gestational age)

Physical examination
- Dx made by visualization or palpation of cord in vagina following premature rupture of membranes
- Fetal bradycardia usually present; may be intrauterine fetal demise

Diagnostic tests
- Cord prolapse clinical Dx; there is no place for ultrasound in acute setting (other than to confirm viable fetus, if indicated)
- Consider cause of rupture of membranes (eg, intraamniotic infection)

DIFFERENTIAL DIAGNOSIS
- Sonographic evidence of umbilical cord in vagina w/ intact membranes defines cord (funic) presentation, not cord prolapse

COMPLICATIONS

- Depends on gestational age, time interval from prolapse to delivery
- In general, prognosis poor, w/ overall perinatal mortality rate >50%
- *Maternal complications* arise from emergent nature of operative delivery
- *Fetal complications:* prematurity, intrauterine fetal distress, ischemic cerebral injury

PROGNOSIS

- Cord prolapse causes immediate decrease in fetal perfusion due to vasospasm or mechanical distortion of cord
- Fetal prognosis dependent on time interval from prolapse to delivery & gestational age

MANAGEMENT

General measures

- Immediate delivery necessary to prevent fetal ischemic injury
- Confirm gestational age (avoid cesarean delivery if fetus previable)

Specific treatment

- Confirm Dx
- Document fetal well-being (usually by pulsation of cord); if cord nonpulsatile, document fetal heart rate
- Immediate manual replacement of cord into uterine cavity (to minimize anatomic distortion & vasospasm)
- Proceed w/ emergent cesarean, usually under general anesthesia
- Practitioner should remove vaginal hand only once baby delivered

Prevention

- Amniotomy only once vertex well applied to cervix

SUBSEQUENT MANAGEMENT
- Recurrence risk unclear & probably related to underlying cause

---

CORTICOSTEROID THERAPY

BACKGROUND
- Assessment of fetal lung maturity rarely indicated <32 wk; most helpful in planning delivery 34–36 wk
- Antenatal corticosteroid Rx increases fetal surfactant (decreases respiratory distress syndrome) & promotes vascular stability in fetus (decreases necrotizing enterocolitis, intraventricular hemorrhage); effect maximal at 48 h & lasts for at least 7 d

DIAGNOSIS

History
- Confirm gestational age
- Identify risk factors for preterm delivery
- Maternal diabetes assoc. w/ delay in fetal lung maturity

Physical examination
- Identify clinical features predictive of preterm delivery

Diagnostic tests
- Ultrasound to confirm gestational age
- Tests suggestive of lung maturity incl. (1) lecithin/sphingomyelin (L/S) ratio >2.1; (2) phosphatidylglycerol >3% of total phospholipid; (3) fluorescence polarization (FLM assay) >=55 mg surfactant/1 g amniotic albumin; (4) lamellar body counts >30,000–40,000/mL amniotic fluid

DIFFERENTIAL DIAGNOSIS
- Transient tachypnea of newborn
- Meconium aspiration
- Pulmonary hypoplasia

COMPLICATIONS

- *Maternal complications:* preterm premature rupture of membranes, bleeding, preterm birth due to amniocentesis; steroid Rx adversely affects glucose control (clinically relevant only in diabetics); no consistent evidence of adrenal suppression, immunosuppression
- *Fetal complications:* no evidence of neonatal compromise w/ 1–2 courses of steroids; >=3 courses association w/ intrauterine growth restriction, smaller head circumference

PROGNOSIS

- Steroid Rx decreases by 50% incidence & severity of respiratory distress syndrome (24–34 wk), intraventricular hemorrhage (24–28 wk), fetal death

MANAGEMENT

General measures

- Indications for fetal lung maturity include planned elective delivery <39 wk, preterm premature rupture of membranes <36 wk
- Corticosteroid Rx recommended for impending preterm delivery <34 wk (<32 wk if preterm premature rupture of membranes)

Specific treatment

- Betamethasone, 12 mg IM q24h × 2 doses or dexamethazone, 6 mg IM q12h × 4 doses (avoid oral dexamethazone because of increased risk of neonatal sepsis)
- Not currently recommended to repeat steroids outside clinical trial; further studies in progress

Contraindications

- Acute infection, need for immediate delivery

Side effects & complications of treatment

- Decrease in fetal activity 24–48 h after steroids

SUBSEQUENT MANAGEMENT
- No known long-term effects of antenatal steroids

CYTOMEGALOVIRUS

BACKGROUND
- Double-stranded DNA herpesvirus
- Transmitted by sexual contact or contact w/ infected blood, saliva, urine, cervicovaginal secretions at birth, or breast milk
- Incidence of primary infection, 0.7–4% pregnancies; recurrent infection, 13.5%

DIAGNOSIS

History
- History of exposure to CMV rare
- Incubation period 40 (28–60) d followed by brief, self-limited, flu-like illness w/ fever, chills, malaise, myalgia, leukocytosis, increased liver function tests
- Majority of infected adults asymptomatic

Physical examination
- Usually unhelpful

Diagnostic tests
- CMV can be detected 2–3 wk after primary infection by culture, polymerase chain reaction preferred
- Dx usually confirmed by serologic testing (seroconversion or >= 4-fold rise in anti-CMV IgG over 4–6 wks); anti-CMV IgM can confirm primary infection but unreliable (sensitivity 50–80%)
- Suspect fetal infection following maternal infection or identification of characteristic structural anomalies on ultrasound; fetal Dx can be confirmed by detection of CMV in amniotic fluid by culture or polymerase chain reaction; percutaneous umbilical cord blood sampling rarely indicated (fetal

serology less sensitive owing to immaturity of fetal immune system)

DIFFERENTIAL DIAGNOSIS
- Other fetal viral or parasitic infections, esp. toxoplasmosis

COMPLICATIONS
- *Maternal complications:* usually mild, self-limiting, flu-like illness; severe complications may develop in immunosuppressed patients (chorioretinitis, encephalitis)
- *Fetal complications:* intrauterine growth restriction, intrauterine fetal demise/neonatal death, ventriculomegaly/hydrocephaly, mental retardation, deafness, chorioretinitis, hydrops fetalis, ascites, hepatosplenomegaly, echogenic bowel, & calcifications in abdomen, liver, & lateral ventricles
- Most infants w/ *congenital CMV* asymptomatic at birth; manifest w/ hepatosplenomegaly, jaundice, petechiae, thrombocytopenia, failure to thrive

PROGNOSIS
- CMV most common congenital infection, occurring in 0.2–2.2% of all neonates
- CMV leading cause of congenital hearing loss
- Structural anomalies, esp. CNS anomalies, associated w/ poor prognosis
- Vertical transmission occurs at any gestational age but most common in 3rd trimester; severe sequelae usually follow 1st trimester transmission
- Overall risk of vertical transmission 30–40% following primary & 0.2–2% following recurrent maternal CMV infection; more severe fetal neurologic sequelae occur following primary infections
- Congenital infection occurs in 40% of cases after primary infection in pregnancy & in 14% of cases after recurrent infection; 85% of infected neonates asymptomatic at birth

MANAGEMENT

General measures
- No effective Rx available; as such, routine serologic screening not recommended in pregnancy

Specific treatment
- Antiretroviral Rx (ganciclovir, foscarnet) used for CMV retinitis in AIDS patients; however, use of ganciclovir in CMV-infected neonates does not prevent neurologic sequelae

SUBSEQUENT MANAGEMENT

Prevention
- Careful handling of potentially infected articles (diapers); meticulous handwashing around young children or immuno-compromised individuals
- Avoid high-risk behavior (IV drug use, unprotected sex); use of barrier contraception
- No vaccine available

Future pregnancies
- Anti-CMV IgG persists for life but does not prevent reinfection
- After initial infection, CMV remains latent & may reactivate; recurrent disease may also be caused by different strain of CMV

DEEP VEIN THROMBOSIS

BACKGROUND
- Venous thromboembolism (VTE) (deep vein thrombosis [DVT] + pulmonary embolism [PE]) occurs in 0.05–0.3% of pregnancies
- Leading obstetric cause of maternal mortality (20–25%)

DIAGNOSIS

History
- May be asymptomatic

- Sx may include leg swelling, pain
- *Risk factors:* pregnancy/puerperium (increases 5-fold), advanced maternal age, multiparity, surgery, bedrest, obesity, inherited thrombophilia

Physical examination
- Often unhelpful
- Signs may include calf tenderness, asymmetric swelling of lower extremities, (+) Homans' sign (50% sensitivity)

Diagnostic tests
- *Laboratory tests:* none
- *Specific diagnostic tests:* none
- *Imaging tests:* lower extremity noninvasive (LENI) ultrasound: more accurate for proximal DVT; definitive Dx by venography
- *Tests to identify cause:* Factor V Leiden mutation (5% of population), G20210A prothrombin (factor II) gene mutation (2%), methylenetetrahydrofolate reductase gene mutation (40% heterozygous, only at risk if homozygous and assoc w/ hyperhomocysteinemia [9%]), antiphospholipid antibody syndrome; deficiency in protein S, protein C, antithrombin III (levels unreliable in pregnancy, esp. protein S)

DIFFERENTIAL DIAGNOSIS
- Pregnancy-related edema
- Preeclampsia

COMPLICATIONS
- *Maternal complications:* PE, maternal mortality; heparin Rx assoc. w/ bleeding, thrombocytopenia, osteoporosis
- *Fetal complications:* prematurity, placental abruption, intrauterine growth restriction, stillbirth; warfarin (Coumadin) teratogenic (not heparin)

PROGNOSIS
- If untreated, 15–25% of women w/ DVT will have PE vs. 4–5% if treated

MANAGEMENT

General measures

■ Treat acute VTE to prevent thrombus propagation, PE

■ Search for predisposing factors, inherited thrombophilia

Specific treatment

■ *Ideal Rx:* unfractionated heparin (UFH) 10,000 U IV/SC tid; check PTT in 2–3 h; titrate to 2.0–2.5× control

■ *Alternative Rx* (less well tested in pregnancy): low-molecular-weight heparin (LMWH) such as enoxaparin (Lovenox) 1 mg/kg q8–12 h, dalteparin (Fragmin) 200 U/kg q8–12 h; consider checking antifactor Xa activity to document therapeutic dosage (0.6–1.0 U/mL); change over to UFH at 35–36 wk because LMWH has long $t^{1}/_{2}$ & is resistant to reversal by protamine sulfate

■ Continue Rx throughout pregnancy & for 6–12 wk postpartum

■ In general, schedule delivery at 39 wk; hold 1–2 doses of UFH (? hold LMWH for >24–28 h); check PTT prior to induction

■ Protamine sulfate (1 mg/100 U heparin, maximum 50 mg in 15 min) reverses UFH but not LMWH

■ *Postpartum:* check PT/PTT; restart IV UFH 6–8 h postpartum × 48 h; start Coumadin (10 mg po qhs × 2 doses) postpartum day 1; adjust Coumadin dose to give INR 1.5–2.0 (Coumadin compatible w/ breastfeeding)

Contraindications

■ Avoid alternative Rx (fibrinolysis, surgery) in pregnancy

Prevention

■ Prophylaxis indicated for history of VTE, prolonged bed rest, high-risk cesarean (decreased mobility, obesity); should be continued during pregnancy & for 6–12 wk postpartum

■ UFH 5,000 U bid SC in 1st trimester, 7,500–10,000 U bid SC in 2nd & 3rd trimesters (don't follow PTT); LMWH: enoxaparin

40 mg or dalteparin 5,000 U SC qd (anti-factor Xa activity 0.1–0.3 U/mL)
- Oral anticoagulation postpartum

SUBSEQUENT MANAGEMENT
- Women w/ history of VTE have 5–12% incidence of recurrence in subsequent pregnancy
- Recurrence rate increased if assoc. w/ inherited thrombophilia
  - Consider evaluation for rheumatologic-connective tissue diseases like systemic lupus erythematosus or antiphospholipid antibody syndrome.

DIABETIC KETOACIDOSIS (DKA)

BACKGROUND
- Characterized by insulin deficiency, hyperglycemia, acidosis
- Incidence in pregnancy: 9% pregestational diabetics, <1% gestational diabetics

DIAGNOSIS

History
- Nausea, vomiting, abdominal pain, polyuria, polydipsia
- *Risk factors:* undiagnosed diabetes, pregnancy, emesis, noncompliance, infection, beta-agonists

Physical examination
- Dehydration: poor tissue turgor, tachycardia, hypotension
- Acidosis: malaise, fatigue, hyperventilation (Kussmaul breathing), coma
- Fruity smell (acetone) on breath

Diagnostic tests
- *Laboratory tests:* check CBC, glucose, electrolytes, ABGs, blood cultures; urinalysis & culture

- *Specific diagnostic tests:* check acetone, ketonuria, ketonemia
- *Imaging:* CXR for pneumonia

5 diagnostic criteria for DKA:

- Glucose >250 mg/dL
- pH <7.30
- Bicarbonate <15 mEq/L
- Anion gap ($Na^\pm$ [$Cl^\mp$ HCO_3-]) >12 mEq/L
- Osmolality ($2[Na^{++}K^+]+[glu/18]$) >280 mOsm/kg

DIFFERENTIAL DIAGNOSIS

- Hyperglycemic coma
- Drug overdose (alcohol)
- Preeclampsia/eclampsia
- Seizure
- Encephalopathy
- Infection
- Uremia
- Psychosis

COMPLICATIONS

- *Maternal complications:* preterm labor, coma, death
- *Fetal complications:* cerebral injury, 35–50% mortality

PROGNOSIS

- Increased maternal/perinatal morbidity & mortality
- Prognosis depends on rapid Dx, Rx

MANAGEMENT

General measures

- Objectives: correct volume deficit, hyperglycemia, electrolyte imbalance, acidosis, Rx precipitating cause

  Note: immediate goal reversal of ketoacidosis, not euglycemia

Specific treatment

- Manage in intensive care setting

- Maternal vital signs q15min
- ECG, O_2 at 4–6 L/min
- Fetal monitoring, if viable
- FLUID: IV N/S 4–5 L over 5 h; $^{1}/_{2}$ NS if Na^+ >155 mEq/L; add 5% dextrose once glucose <250 mg/dL
- INSULIN: 10 U regular IV push then 6 U/h (0.1 U/kg/h) in N/S; check serum glucose hourly (should decrease to 60 mg/dL/h); stop insulin for 1 h if glucose <80 mg/dL; restart subcutaneous insulin once patient eating
- POTASSIUM: 10–40 mEq KCl per liter to maintain K^+ 4–5 mEq/L; check K+ hourly; stop if >5.5 mEq/L, oliguria
- BICARB: if pH <7.0, consider 2 amp (88 mEq) $NaHCO_3$ in 1 L N/S over 1 h, repeat as needed
- Antibiotics, if indicated

SUBSEQUENT MANAGEMENT
- Prevent DKA: patient education, frequent visits, rigorous glycemic control

---

ECLAMPSIA

BACKGROUND
- Refers to generalized convulsions or coma in setting of pre-eclampsia & in absence of other neurologic conditions
- Eclampsia was thought to be end point of preeclampsia (hence the nomenclature) but is probably one manifestation of severe preeclampsia
- 50% of eclampsia occurs preterm; of those cases at term, 75% occur intrapartum or w/in 48 h of delivery

DIAGNOSIS
History
- Witnessed generalized convulsion
- Seizures preceded by prodromal sx (headache, visual changes) in 70% of cases

Physical examination

■ Check BP, proteinuria, urine output (although 20% of eclamptic women have maximum BP <140/90 mmHg &/or proteinuria <300 mg/d before seizure)

■ Evaluate maternal neurologic & hemodynamic status; check for focal neurologic signs (confusion, hyperreflexia, positive Babinski sign may be consistent w/ postictal state)

Diagnostic tests

■ Eclampsia a *clinical* Dx

■ Evaluate for other complications of severe preeclampsia (thrombocytopenia, HELLP syndrome [hemolysis, elevated liver enzymes, low platelets], pulmonary edema, renal failure, cardiac failure)

■ If focal neurologic signs develop or seizures persist, consider head CT to exclude intracranial hemorrhage

DIFFERENTIAL DIAGNOSIS

■ Idiopathic seizure disorder (epilepsy)

■ Drug withdrawal (alcohol, cocaine)

■ Intracranial pathology (hemorrhage, tumor)

COMPLICATIONS

■ *Maternal complications:* intracranial hemorrhage (usually assoc w/ BP > = 170/120 mmHg), placental abruption, other complications of severe preeclampsia, maternal mortality

■ *Fetal complications:* bradycardia, acute uteroplacental insufficiency & possible neurologic injury, stillbirth

PROGNOSIS

■ Eclamptic seizures classically last 2–3 min & resolve spontaneously; if seizures persist, consider intracranial hemorrhage

■ Preeclampsia & its complications always resolve following delivery (w/ exception of stroke)

■ Fetal prognosis depends largely on gestational age at delivery & problems related to prematurity

MANAGEMENT

General measures

- Eclampsia a contraindication to expectant management of severe preeclampsia; immediate delivery indicated
- Although there is no proven benefit to routine cesarean delivery, the probability of vaginal delivery in patient w/ severe preeclampsia remote from term w/ an unfavorable cervix is only 14–20%
- BP control important to prevent stroke but does not affect course of preeclampsia or prevent eclampsia

Specific treatment

- Protect airway, establish IV access
- Check CBC, type & screen
- Anesthesia consult
- Continuous fetal monitoring: fetal heart rate usually decreases to 60–80 bpm for 6–8 min following seizure & then resolves spontaneously
- Attempt to resuscitate fetus in utero before proceeding w/ delivery
- Because seizures are short-lived, IV diazepam rarely indicated to terminate seizures (& may lead to further neonatal depression)
- Start IV magnesium sulfate seizure prophylaxis (6 g loading dose over 20–30 min, 2 g/h infusion intrapartum & for at least 24 h postpartum); follow w/ hourly neurologic exams (incl. deep tendon reflexes) or serum magnesium levels q6h (keep levels at 4–8 mg/dL)
- Magnesium will not prevent all seizures; if seizures persist, consider adding second agent (diazepam, phenytoin)

Complications of therapy

- Magnesium overdose (serum levels $> = 12$ mg/dL) assoc. w/ cardiorespiratory arrest

SUBSEQUENT MANAGEMENT
- Eclampsia not a risk factor for seizures in later life
- 2–10% recurrence rate of eclampsia in subsequent pregnancy

ENDOMYOMETRITIS

BACKGROUND
- Refers to infection w/in uterine cavity following delivery
- Complicates 6–8% of deliveries
- Most infections polymicrobial; single-agent infections more common after vaginal delivery; anaerobic pathogens more common after cesarean

DIAGNOSIS

History
- Chills, malaise, lower abdominal discomfort following delivery
- *Risk factors:* diabetes, prolonged premature rupture of membranes (risk inversely proportional to latency), uterine instrumentation, cesarean

Physical examination
- Fever, abdominal tenderness (esp. tenderness over uterine fundus), foul lochia

Diagnostic tests
- Endomyometritis a *clinical* Dx
- Check blood cultures, CBC
- Culture of endometrial cavity not routinely recommended
- Imaging studies not routinely indicated (may be useful to exclude retained tissue, septic thrombophlebitis)

DIFFERENTIAL DIAGNOSIS
- Retained products of conception
- Septic thrombophlebitis

- Appendicitis
- Pyelonephritis
- Pneumonia
- Pelvic/bladder flap hematoma
- Wound infection

COMPLICATIONS
- *Maternal complications:* sepsis, necrotizing fasciitis, subsequent Asherman syndrome (esp. w/ uterine instrumentation)
- *Fetal complications:* not applicable

PROGNOSIS
- Prognosis good w/ early & adequate Rx

MANAGEMENT
General measures
- Inpatient Rx recommended
- Cooling, antipyretic Rx as needed

Specific treatment
- Appropriate Rx: (1) penicillin & aminoglycoside after vaginal delivery; (2) gentamicin 1.5 mg/kg plus clindamycin 900 mg IV q8h after cesarean (substitute aztreonam for gentamicin if abscess suspected or renal impairment develops)
- Continue IV Rx until 24–48 h afebrile, asymptomatic
- 10% fail to respond w/in 48–72 h; 20% due to resistant organisms; consider adding ampicillin for enterococcal coverage, evaluate for other source of infection

Side effects & complications of treatment
- Pseudomembranous colitis may develop w/ prolonged antibiotic Rx

Prevention
- Avoid frequent vaginal exams, uterine instrumentation (incl. manual removal of placenta at cesarean)

■ Prophylaxis w/ cephalosporin (or clindamycin/gentamicin) for cesarean decreases wound infection, endometritis

SUBSEQUENT MANAGEMENT
■ No role for oral antibiotics once discharged (aside from pts w/ proven bacteremia who require 10–14 d of antibiotics)

EPISIOTOMY

BACKGROUND
■ Surgical incision made in perineum to facilitate vaginal delivery
■ Introduced to decrease complications of pelvic floor trauma at delivery; however, no proven benefit to elective (prophylactic) episiotomy
■ Still performed in 30–50% of nulliparous vaginal deliveries in U.S.

DIAGNOSIS

History and physical examination
■ History of prior episiotomies & complications
■ Risk factors: nulliparity, assisted vaginal delivery, fetal macrosomia, prior episiotomy, epidural analgesia, prolonged second stage of labor, obstetric care provider preference

Diagnostic tests
■ Anal endosonography, manometry can identify anal sphincter injury in up to 35% of vaginal deliveries even in absence of perineal laceration but not routinely used

DIFFERENTIAL DIAGNOSIS
■ By definition, episiotomy is 2nd degree perineal laceration

COMPLICATIONS

■ *Short-term maternal complications:* extension of episiotomy into external anal sphincter (3rd & 4th perineal lacerations), pain, bleeding, infection, hematoma, episiotomy breakdown, edema

■ *Long-term maternal complications:* urinary/fecal incontinence, rectovaginal fistulas, genital prolapse, cosmetic deformity, dyspareunia (?)

■ *Fetal complications:* trauma (rare)

PROGNOSIS

■ Despite location, most episiotomies heal w/o incident

MANAGEMENT

General measures

■ No proven maternal or fetal benefits to routine (prophylactic) episiotomy, aside from decrease in anterior perineal lacerations

■ No absolute indication for episiotomy

■ Legitimate indications include nonreassuring fetal testing, assisted vaginal delivery, & shoulder dystocia (extreme prematurity, suspected fetal macrosomia not acceptable indications)

Specific treatment

■ Confirm indication for episiotomy

■ Select midline (median), mediolateral, or modified median (J-shape) episiotomy: midline incision assoc. w/ increased incidence of severe perineal trauma; unclear whether mediolateral incision protects against anal sphincter injury; mediolateral episiotomy may be assoc. w/ increased blood loss, pain (not proven)

■ Ensure adequate analgesia (local field block, pudendal, regional)

■ Cut episiotomy w/ contraction

Follow-up care

- After delivery, examine perineum for extension of episiotomy into anal sphincter &/or rectum; failure to correctly identify & repair such an extension increases probability of postpartum complications
- Primary approximation affords best opportunity for functional repair, esp. if rectal sphincter involvement
- External anal sphincter best repaired by overlapping cut ends & securing them using interrupted absorbable sutures; such repairs should be effected by experienced obstetric care providers, not junior staff members
- Perform rectal exam after repair to ensure that no sutures were placed through the rectal mucosa (may predispose to rectovaginal fistula)
- Ice to perineum for 24 h to minimize swelling; thereafter, keep perineum clean & dry using sitzbaths
- Adequate pain management
- Avoid constipation in immediate postpartum period through use of bulking agents, stool softeners
- No proven benefit to routine antibiotic therapy

SUBSEQUENT MANAGEMENT

Prevention

- Avoid routine episiotomy
- If indicated, consider mediolateral episiotomy to minimize anal sphincter injury

Subsequent pregnancy

- Prior episiotomy a risk factor for episiotomy at subsequent delivery
- Vaginal delivery carries inherent risk to perineum, which may not become apparent until many years later; unclear whether episiotomy modifies this risk

FETAL BRADYARRHYTHMIA

BACKGROUND
- Defined as sustained fetal heart rate <110 bpm
- May be assoc. w/ fetal acidemia, hypoxemia
- *Classification:*
  1. Complete heart block: 1/20,000 pregnancies, 50% due to maternal autoimmune disease; also assoc. w/ structural heart disease
  2. 2nd degree heart block: can progress to complete block, esp. if assoc. w/ autoimmune disease

DIAGNOSIS

History
- *Risk factors:* maternal connective tissue disease (SLE, Sjogren syndrome), thyroid dysfunction, antiphospholipid antibody syndrome

Physical examination
- Evidence of connective tissue diseases (Raynaud's, malar rash)

Diagnostic tests
- *Laboratory tests:* check anti-Ro (Sjogren syndrome antigen A, SS-A), anti-La (Sjogren syndrome antigen B, SS-B)
- *Specific diagnostic tests:* offer amniocentesis for karyotype if structural anomaly
- *Imaging tests:* ultrasound to assess fetal cardiac/CNS anatomy, amniotic fluid volume, hydrops; M-mode to determine rhythm disturbance (atrial bigeminy, sinus bradycardia, 2nd degree or complete heart block)
- *Screening tests:* check fetal heart rate & rhythm each prenatal visit

DIFFERENTIAL DIAGNOSIS

- Uteroplacental deficiency (cord prolapse, cord compression, uterine contractions, abruption)
- Maternal antithyroid antibodies
- Complex congenital heart defect
- Fetal CNS anomaly, malformation

COMPLICATIONS

- *Maternal complications:* none
- *Fetal complications:* hydrops, intrauterine growth restriction, intrauterine fetal demise

PROGNOSIS

- Prognosis better in absence of congenital cardiac anomaly

MANAGEMENT

General measures

- Manage at tertiary care center w/ pediatric cardiology backup
- Antenatal corticosteroids for usual obstetric indications

Specific treatment

- Ultrasound q wk for hydrops
- >34 wk, check atrial rate (slowing of atrial rate suggests fetal compromise)
- In absence of hydrops, deliver at favorable gestational age or once fetal lung maturity confirmed
- If hydrops, consider immediate delivery; if <32 wk w/ hydrops & maternal autoimmune disease, consider dexamethazone Rx
- Cesarean delivery often recommended because intrapartum fetal monitoring difficult

Follow-up care

- Neonates may require cardiac pacemaker

SUBSEQUENT MANAGEMENT
- Consider rheumatologic follow-up
- 8% recurrence rate if assoc. w/ maternal autoimmune disease; often occurs earlier in successive pregnancies

---

FETAL LABORATORY VALUES

TABLES
- Normal fetal lab values are affected by gestational age

Hematologic Tests		Gestational Age		
Values (mean)	<22	22–25	26–30	>30
WBC (k/mm^3)	4.7	4.7	5.2	7.7
Plts (k/mm^3)	234	247	242	232
HCT (%)	37	39	41	44
Hgb (g/dL)	12	12	13	14
MCV (fl)	131	125	118	114

Serum Chemistry		Gestational Age		
Values (mean)	<22	22–25	26–30	>30
Na$^+$(mEq/L)	136	135	136	135
K$^+$(mEq/L)	3.6	3.5	3.6	3.5
Cr (mg/dL)	41	42	42	45
BUN (mg/dL)	3.2	3.4	3.0	3.3
Ca^{++} (mg/dL)	2.2	2.2	2.3	2.3
PO$_4$(mg/dL)	1.13	1.15	1.13	1.10
Albumin (g/dL)	18	23	29	32
T. bili (mg/L)	15.5	16.5	18.5	18.5
AST (U/L)	16	20	20	26
ALP (U/L)	246	251	234	204

FETAL pH			Gestational Age	
Values (mean)	22	28	34	40
Umb vein	7.416	7.407	7.398	7.388
Umb artery	7.390	9.379	7.368	7.357

FETAL PO			Gestational Age	
Values (mean, mmHg)	22	28	34	40
Umb. vein	47.6	42.0	36.3	30.6
Umb. artery	28.3	26.3	24.3	22.3

FETAL PCO_2			Gestational Age	
Values (mean, mmHg)	22	28	34	40
Umb. vein	33.6	34.9	36.2	37.5

FETAL HCO_3			Gestational Age	
Values (mean, mEq/L)	22	28	34	40
Umb. vein	22.3	23.0	23.7	24.3

FETAL TACHYARRHYTHMIA

BACKGROUND
- Sustained fetal heart rate >180 bpm
- *Etiology:* supraventricular tachycardia (SVT; 0.5% of pregnancies), atrial flutter, ventricular & sinus tachycardia

DIAGNOSIS
History
- Usually asymptomatic
- May have nonspecific sx (malaise, contractions, abdominal pain)

Physical examination
- Uterine tenderness, contractions
- Evidence of hyperthyroidism (goiter, maternal tachycardia, tremor, hyperreflexia)

Diagnostic tests
- *Laboratory tests:* check CBC, thyroid-stimulating hormone
- *Specific diagnostic tests:* consider amniocentesis to exclude chorioamnionitis
- *Imaging tests:* ultrasound to assess fetal cardiac/CNS anatomy, hydrops; M-mode echocardiogram to determine rhythm disturbance:
  - ➤ SVT: 200 bpm, 1:1 conduction
  - ➤ Atrial flutter: 400 bpm, 2:1 block
  - ➤ Sinus tachycardia: 200 bpm, 1:1 conduction
- *Screening:* check fetal heart rate & rhythm each prenatal visit

DIFFERENTIAL DIAGNOSIS
- Uteroplacental insufficiency
- Maternal Graves' disease
- Complex congenital heart defect
- Maternal infection, fever
- Chorioamnionitis

COMPLICATIONS
- *Maternal complications:* rare
- *Fetal complications:* hydrops, intrauterine fetal demise

PROGNOSIS
- Prognosis poor once hydrops develops
- Hydrops likely if tachycardia sustained >48 h; normalization of fetal heart rate decreases risk of hydrops

MANAGEMENT
General measures
- Mx at tertiary care center w/ pediatric cardiology backup

- Antenatal corticosteroids for usual obstetric indications

Specific treatment
- Ultrasound q wk for hydrops
- Rx of sinus tachycardia secondary to maternal infection: IV antibiotics, Rx infection, deliver for chorioamnionitis
- If tachycardia sustained >48 h, consider delivery if gestational age favorable or fetal lung maturity confirmed; if remote from term, consider maternal digoxin Rx
- Vaginal delivery not contraindicated; continuous intrapartum fetal monitoring recommended

Side effects & complications of treatment
- Digoxin toxicity in mother
- Maternal cardiac arrhythmia

SUBSEQUENT MANAGEMENT
- Recurrence sporadic & nonspecific; depends on cause

GESTATIONAL DIABETES

BACKGROUND
- Pregnancy a "diabetogenic" state due to placental anti-insulin hormones that ensure continuous supply of glucose for fetus
- Gestational diabetes mellitus (GDM) refers to abnormal handling of glucose during pregnancy
- Complicates 3–5% of pregnancies

DIAGNOSIS
History
- Asymptomatic
- May have personal history of GDM, prior macrosomic infant, or family history of diabetes

➤ High-risk ethnic groups: Asian, Native American, African American

➤ High-risk foods include reliance on carbohydrates, particularly processed rice in diet

Physical examination
- Not helpful

Diagnostic tests
- Glucose load test (GLT) screening recommended for all pregnant women at 24–28 wk; consider early screening (16–20 wk) in women w/ sustained glycosuria, obesity, family history of diabetes, or history of GDM, unexplained intrauterine fetal demise, fetal macrosomia
- GLT is a nonfasting test to assess the woman's ability to handle a 50-g glucose load over 1 h; $> = 140$ mg/dL is considered positive (this cutoff detects 80% of women w/ GDM with a 15% false-positive rate).
- Definitive Dx requires glucose tolerance test (GTT): 100-g glucose load after overnight fast & plasma glucose measured fasting & at 1 h, 2 h, & 3 h (GDM requires 2 or more abnormal values defined by NDDG as $> = 105$, $> = 190$, $> = 165$, & $> = 145$ mg/dL, respectively)

DIFFERENTIAL DIAGNOSIS
- Pregestational diabetes
- Isolated glucosuria (due to increased renal clearance of glucose in pregnancy) w/o GDM

COMPLICATIONS
- *Maternal complications:* maternal risk small (such women *not* at risk of diabetic ketoacidosis); increased risk of cesarean
- *Fetal complications:* fetal macrosomia leading to increased risk of birth injury

PROGNOSIS

- Fetal complications related to ability to maintain strict glycemic control & prevent fetal macrosomia
- GDM typically resolves after delivery

MANAGEMENT

General measures

- Goal: to prevent fetal macrosomia & its complications by maintaining blood glucose at desirable levels in pregnancy (fasting, <95 mg/dL; 1 h postprandial <140 mg/dL; 2 h postprandial, <120 mg/dL)
- Diabetic diet recommended for all women w/ GDM
- If diet alone fails to maintain blood glucose at desirable levels, insulin may be required (if fasting glucose levels are >105 mg/dL, insulin can be initiated right away)
- Oral hypoglycemic agents best avoided in pregnancy until further data are available, although recent studies suggest they may be safe and effective

Specific treatment

- Weekly follow-up & evaluation of qid glucose monitoring
- Adjustment of insulin therapy, if indicated
- Ultrasound for estimated fetal weight at 36–37 wk
- Timing of delivery for GDM controversial; consider increased fetal monitoring after 34 wks with delivery by 40 wks
- Elective cesarean may be indicated if estimated fetal weight excessive (> = 4,500 g) because of risk of birth injury
- In labor, maintain blood glucose at 100–120 mg/dL
- Since main source of anti-insulin hormones is placenta, no further Mx required in immediate postpartum period
- Check neonatal blood glucose level w/in 1 h of birth

Complications of treatment

- Iatrogenic hypoglycemia due to excessive insulin administration

SUBSEQUENT MANAGEMENT

Prevention
- GDM cannot be prevented

Maternal implications
- GDM good screening test for insulin resistance: 50% of women develop GDM in subsequent pregnancy, & 40–60% develop diabetes later in life
- All women w/ GDM should have standard (nonpregnant) 75-g GTT 6–8 wk postpartum

---

GONORRHEA

BACKGROUND
- 2nd most common sexually transmitted disease (STD) in U.S.
- Incidence: <1–7% of pregnancies, depending on population
- 5-d incubation period from exposure to sx

DIAGNOSIS

History
- Frequently asymptomatic
- Sx may include vaginal, anal, pharyngeal pain; dysuria
- *Risk factors:* multiple sexual partners, young age, concurrent STD (incl. HIV), partners of men w/ urethritis, IV drug abuse

Physical examination
- Frequently unhelpful
- Purulent cervical discharge, anal/pharyngeal lesions, urethral discharge
- *Disseminated infection:* stage 1 characterized by fever, chills, small pustular skin lesion w/ hemorrhagic base & center necrosis; stage 2 pts have arthritis (knees, wrists, ankles) w/ purulent synovial fluid

Diagnostic tests

- *Laboratory tests:* check cervical ELISA, stain (Gram stain only 60% positive predictive value)
- *Specific diagnostic tests:* cervical culture on Thayer-Martin medium in CO_2-enriched environment; blood culture if suspect disseminated disease
- *Imaging tests:* not routinely indicated
- *Screening tests:* check cervical ELISA in 1st trimester, repeat in 3rd trimester if high risk

DIFFERENTIAL DIAGNOSIS

- HIV infection
- Chlamydia infection
- Syphilis
- Nonspecific cervicitis

COMPLICATIONS

- *Maternal complications:* increased preterm premature rupture of membranes, disseminated infection in pregnancy
- *Fetal complications:* gonococcal ophthalmia neonatorum; chorioamnionitis rare (but may occur w/ preterm premature rupture of membranes)

PROGNOSIS

- Infection curable if compliant w/ Rx
- Consider resistant organism if infection persists

MANAGEMENT

General measures

- Screen for concurrent STDs

Specific treatment

- Antibiotic Rx: cefuroxime, 400 mg po × 1 or ceftriaxone, 125 mg IM × 1

- Consider treating also for presumed concurrent infection w/ *Chlamydia trachomatis:* amoxicillin, 500 mg po tid × 7 d or azithromycin, 1 g po × 1

Contraindications
- Penicillin allergy: use spectinomycin, 2 g IM × 1
- Quinolones contraindicated in pregnancy (CNS side effects)

Follow-up care
- Obtain test of cure 2–3 wk after Rx

SUBSEQUENT MANAGEMENT
- Evaluate according to risk factors

GROUP B STREPTOCOCCUS

BACKGROUND
- Group B beta-hemolytic streptococcus (GBS), or *Streptococcus agalactiae*, is leading cause of perinatal infection in U.S. (>8,000 cases/y)
- Incidence 1–3/1,000 term births; 40–50/1,000 preterm births
- 80% of neonatal GBS infection early onset (acquired at delivery & develops w/in 7 d of birth)
- GBS colonizes lower genital/GI tract of 20% of pregnant women but not same 20% throughout pregnancy (8–10% crossover in carrier status each trimester)

DIAGNOSIS

History
- Parturient usually asymptomatic
- Prior urinary tract infection

Physical examination
- Unhelpful in mother
- Early-onset neonatal GBS infection presents as respiratory distress, apnea, pneumonia w/in 7 d of birth; late-onset GBS manifests after 7 d, usually as sepsis/meningitis

Diagnostic tests
- Dx of neonatal GBS sepsis requires positive blood culture
- Women colonized w/ GBS identified by perineal and perianal (not cervical or vaginal) culture using selective broth media; results are reliable for 5 wks; culture at 35–37 wk accurately reflects GBS carrier status at delivery

DIFFERENTIAL DIAGNOSIS
- Other causes of neonatal sepsis

COMPLICATIONS
- *Maternal complications:* chorioamnionitis, UTI
- *Fetal complications:* intrauterine fetal demise/neonatal death, preterm birth, neonatal sepsis

PROGNOSIS
- 50% of infants born to colonized women will themselves be colonized but most asymptomatic
- Early-onset neonatal GBS infection has mortality rate of 5% (>25% in preterm infants)

MANAGEMENT

General measures
- Intrapartum (but not antepartum) chemoprophylaxis shown to decrease early-onset neonatal GBS infection; does not change the rate of late-onset neonatal GBS infection (which is a hospital-acquired disease)
- Women who had GBS bacteriuria in the index pregnancy or a prior GBS-infected infant should all receive intrapartum chemoprophylaxis; no perineal/perianal culture is required.
- U.S. Centers for Disease Control & Prevention recommends that all other pregnant women have their GBS colonization status documented by perineal/perianal culture at 35–37 wks. GBS(+) women should receive intrapartum chemoprophylaxis. GBS(−) women should receive antibiotics in labor only

if they have a risk factor for early-onset GBS sepsis (prolonged rupture of membranes [>=18 h] or fever in labor).

■ Culture-based protocol will Rx 15–20% of pregnant women & prevent 70–80% of early-onset neonatal GBS disease.

■ Women with unknown GBS status in labor should receive intrapartum chemoprophylaxis only if they have 1 or more risk factors for early-onset GBS sepsis–ie, preterm labor, prolonged rupture of membranes (>=18 h), or fever in labor (which requires broad-spectrum antibiotics).

Specific treatment

■ Intrapartum GBS chemoprophylaxis w/ IV penicillin; alternatives include ampicillin, clindamycin, erythromycin, vancomycin

■ Minimum of 4 h of penicillin recommended prior to delivery, minimum exposure for other antibiotics unclear

■ Antibiotic prophylaxis should be discontinued at delivery; only pts w/ chorioamnionitis require Rx beyond delivery

Prevention

■ Intrapartum GBS chemoprophylaxis for all pregnancies at risk (above)

■ Currently no GBS vaccine

Side effects & complications of treatment

■ Antibiotic resistance (15–20% for erythromycin and clindamycin) & increased neonatal sepsis due to non-GBS organisms

■ Maternal anaphylaxis (1:60,000 for penicillin)

SUBSEQUENT MANAGEMENT

■ GBS colonization in 1 pregnancy not a risk factor for early-onset neonatal GBS sepsis in subsequent pregnancy

HEADACHE

BACKGROUND

■ Common complaint in pregnancy

- Incidence: 20–25% of all pregnancies
- Majority benign; headaches that disturb sleep, exertional in nature, or assoc. w/ focal neurologic findings may indicate underlying structural lesion

DIAGNOSIS

History

- Ask about headaches prior to pregnancy, recent spinal anesthesia
- Note onset, severity, location, timing, radiation of pain, & precipitating, relieving factors; headaches that disturb sleep or exertional in nature require further investigation
- Ask about depressive sx

Physical examination

- Usually unhelpful
- Exclude preeclampsia (check BP, proteinuria), meningitis (nuchal rigidity), sinusitis (facial tenderness), temporal arteritis (focal tenderness over temporal artery)

Diagnostic tests

- *Laboratory tests:* none indicated
- *Specific diagnostic tests:* exclude other Dx (lumbar puncture for pressure, meningitis)
- *Imaging:* consider head CT or MRI to exclude structural lesion

DIFFERENTIAL DIAGNOSIS

- Common causes include tension headache, migraine, depression
- Less common causes include severe preeclampsia, pseudotumor cerebri (benign intracranial hypertension), cerebrovascular disease, hematoma, sinusitis, cerebral tumors, temporal arteritis (giant cell arteritis), infection (meningitis, encephalitis), spinal headache, drug withdrawal

COMPLICATIONS

- *Maternal complications:* pain leading to maternal incapacitation

■ *Fetal complications:* related to underlying cause, complications of Rx

PROGNOSIS
■ Related to underlying cause

MANAGEMENT
General measures
■ Exclude preeclampsia, intracranial structural lesion
■ Adequate pain control
■ Remove trigger factors for migraine (eg, caffeine, chocolate)
■ Antibiotics for sinusitis, meningitis

Specific treatment
■ Immediate delivery if headache occurs in setting of preeclampsia
■ Spinal headache occurs in 30% of women w/in a week of spinal analgesia, usually mild & self-limiting; epidural blood patch may accelerate resolution

Contraindications
■ Ergotamine to abort migraine contraindicated in pregnancy (potential adverse effect on uteroplacental perfusion)
■ Avoid sumatriptan (Imitrex) in pregnancy (limited data)

Follow-up care
■ Regular (weekly) follow-up

SUBSEQUENT MANAGEMENT
■ Depends on cause
■ Successive pregnancies may have similar pattern of migraine exacerbation

HEPATITIS B

BACKGROUND
■ Small DNA virus

- Clinical relevant antigens: surface antigen (HBsAg) on viral surface & free in serum; core antigen (HBcAg) in hepatocytes; envelope antigen (HBeAg) only expressed w/ high viral load
- Acute hepatitis B occurs in 1/1,000 pregnancies; chronic hepatitis B in 10/1,000 pregnancies

DIAGNOSIS

History
- Frequently asymptomatic
- May have fever, malaise, fatigue, nausea, RUQ pain
- *Risk factors:* multiple sexual partners, household or occupational exposure (esp. hemodialysis unit), IV drug abuse, prior blood transfusion, chronically hospitalized

Physical examination
- Frequently unhelpful
- Check for jaundice, RUQ tenderness

Diagnostic tests
- *Laboratory tests:* check transaminase levels, bilirubin, coagulation profile
- *Specific diagnostic tests:* check HBsAg, HBcAg, HBeAg
- *Imaging tests:* not indicated
- *Screening tests:* check HBsAg routinely in early pregnancy

DIFFERENTIAL DIAGNOSIS
- Hepatitis A, C, D
- Cytomegalovirus hepatitis
- Pancreatitis
- Gallbladder disease
- HELLP (hemolysis, elevated liver enzymes, low platelets) syndrome, preeclampsia
- Acute fatty liver of pregnancy
- Cholestasis of pregnancy

COMPLICATIONS
- *Maternal complications:* cirrhosis, hepatocellular carcinoma
- *Fetal complications:* neonatal infection

PROGNOSIS
- Vertical transmission related to maternal status (10–20% if HBsAg-positive, 90% if HBeAg-positive) & gestational age (10% if infected in 1st trimester, 90% in 3rd trimester)
- 85% of infected individuals clear infection & develop protective antibodies; 15% chronically infected w/ detectable HBsAg but have normal hepatic function; 15% chronically infected w/ persistent viral replication, HBeAg expression

MANAGEMENT
General measures
- Hospitalize for acute infection w/ encephalopathy, coagulopathy
- No Rx available in pregnancy once infected

Specific treatment
- Hepatitis B vaccine in pregnancy for patients at high risk
- Following exposure, immunize & Rx w/ hepatitis B immune globulin (HBIG) 0.06 mL/kg

Contraindications
- Interferon-alpha contraindicated in pregnancy

Follow-up care
- Exposed neonates should receive HBIG by 12 h, hepatitis B vaccine by 6 mo of life

SUBSEQUENT MANAGEMENT
- Check hepatic function in subsequent pregnancies

HEPATITIS C

BACKGROUND
- Single-stranded RNA virus
- Incidence: 6/1,000 pregnancies
- 6 genotypes of HCV known; type Ib most severe & least likely to respond to Rx

DIAGNOSIS

History
- Frequently asymptomatic
- May have fever, malaise, fatigue, nausea, RUQ pain
- *Risk factors:* multiple sexual partners, household or occupational exposure (esp. hemodialysis unit), IV drug abuse, prior blood transfusion, chronically hospitalized

Physical examination
- Frequently unhelpful
Check for jaundice, RUQ tenderness

Diagnostic tests
- *Laboratory tests:* check transaminase levels, bilirubin, coagulation profile
- *Specific diagnostic tests:* check HCV antibody test (may take 3 mo to become positive after acute infection), HCV RNA level
- *Imaging tests:* not indicated
- *Screening tests:* routine screening for HBsAg (not HCV) in early pregnancy

DIFFERENTIAL DIAGNOSIS
- Hepatitis A, B, D
- Cytomegalovirus hepatitis
- Pancreatitis
- Gallbladder disease

- HELLP (hemolysis, elevated liver enzymes, low platelets) syndrome, preeclampsia
- Acute fatty liver of pregnancy
- Cholestasis of pregnancy

COMPLICATIONS
- *Maternal complications:* cirrhosis, hepatocellular carcinoma
- *Fetal complications:* neonatal infection

PROGNOSIS
- Vertical transmission 5–8%, but increased if pt HIV-positive, high maternal serum viral load
- Among acutely infected individuals, 50% progress to chronic liver disease; 20% develop chronic active hepatitis w/ increased risk of cirrhosis

MANAGEMENT

General measures
- Hospitalize for acute infection w/ encephalopathy, coagulopathy
- No Rx available in pregnancy once infected

Specific treatment
- No current antibody or vaccine prophylaxis available
- No evidence of decreased transmission w/ cesarean over vaginal delivery

Contraindications
- Interferon-alpha contraindicated in pregnancy
- Breastfeeding controversial w/ chronic hepatitis C infection (<3% risk of transmission to neonate)

Follow-up care
- No effective vaccine available for exposed neonates
- Long-term follow-up w/ gastroenterology, hepatology studies

SUBSEQUENT MANAGEMENT

- Check hepatic function in subsequent pregnancies

HERPES SIMPLEX VIRUS

BACKGROUND

- Caused by member of Herpesviridae family of DNA viruses, known as herpes simplex virus (HSV)
- Two major serotypes, HSV-1 (causes conjunctivitis, stomatitis, gingivitis; 20% of genital infection) & HSV-2 (80% of genital infection)
- Common viral pathogen in U.S. w/ >45 million infected, >500,000 new cases/y, ~30% of women have antibodies to HSV-2
- 1,500–2,000 cases of neonatal HSV/y in U.S.; most due to HSV-2

DIAGNOSIS

History

- History of recent exposure to HSV
- History of prior HSV suggests recurrent infection

Physical examination

- Depends on stage of infection:
  a. *First episode primary* refers to first clinical presentation & absence of anti-HSV IgG; painful vesicles appear on vulva, vagina, cervix 2–14 d after exposure w/ tender adenopathy & systemic sx in 2/3 of cases; lesions resolve in 3–4 wk w/out Rx
  b. *First episode nonprimary* refers to first clinical presentation & presence of anti-HSV IgG
  c. *Recurrent* infection refers to reactivation of dormant virus; sx generally less severe

Diagnostic tests
- Viral isolation from vesicular fluid, infected tissues can confirm Dx but specimen sampling & transporting difficulties limit sensitivity to 60–70%
- Serologic tests do not easily distinguish between anti-HSV-1 & anti-HSV-2 antibodies

DIFFERENTIAL DIAGNOSIS
- Other herpesvirus infections, such as varicella zoster

COMPLICATIONS
- *Maternal complications:* hepatitis, encephalitis, death
- *Fetal complications:* preterm birth, intrauterine fetal demise/neonatal mortality (15–60%), localized (skin, eye, mouth, CNS) or disseminated HSV

PROGNOSIS
- First episode primary infection leads to viremia & increased risk of vertical transmission; however, in utero infection rare
- Most neonatal infections result from contact w/ infected secretions at vaginal delivery; neonatal disease occurs in 30–60% of infants exposed to HSV at vaginal delivery
- Recurrent HSV not assoc. w/ viremia; fetus not at risk if fetal membranes intact & there is no labor

MANAGEMENT

General measures
- Screen for other sexually transmitted diseases
- Confirm Dx
- To prevent vertical transmission, cesarean delivery recommended for active lesion or clinical prodrome in labor

Specific treatment
- Antiviral Rx of first episode primary HSV can decrease severity & duration of sx in mother but does not prevent fetal infection
- Topical less effective than oral Rx & not recommended

- Acyclovir Rx of choice; alternatives include valacyclovir, famciclovir
- Rx disseminated disease w/ IV acyclovir
- Unclear whether antiviral Rx decreases severity or duration of sx in recurrent HSV; may abort outbreak but only if given during clinical prodrome or <1 d of onset of lesions
- Follow fetus w/ serial ultrasound

Prevention
- Avoid contact w/ infected persons
- Use of barrier contraception
- Due to low yield of viral cultures & poor correlation between culture & asymptomatic viral shedding in labor, screening for viral shedding not recommended
- Antiviral prophylaxis from 35–36 wk recommended for women at risk of viral shedding at delivery (incl. first episode genital HSV in index pregnancy & frequent recurrences >12/y) to decrease cesarean delivery rate & (possibly) vertical transmission
- No vaccine available

SUBSEQUENT MANAGEMENT
- Anti-HSV-1 IgG does not prevent primary infection w/ HSV-2, & vice versa

---

HUMAN IMMUNODEFICIENCY VIRUS (HIV)

BACKGROUND
- Vertical transmission rate w/o Rx 25–33%
- Risk of transmission highest during labor, delivery
- Zidovudine (AZT) Rx throughout pregnancy, labor, & to neonate for 6 wk decreases transmission to 8%
- Viral load <1,000 copies/mL decreases transmission to <2%

■ AZT & elective cesarean before labor decrease transmission to <1% (range, 0–2%)

DIAGNOSIS

History
■ Ask about sexually transmitted diseases (STDs), opportunistic infections, cervical dysplasia/cancer
■ *Risk factors:* STDs, drug abuse, prostitution, blood transfusion before 1985, HIV-positive/bisexual partner

Physical examination
■ Usually asymptomatic
■ Nonspecific sx (weight loss, skin lesions)
■ Exam may reveal thrush, chronic vaginitis, cervical lesion, generalized lymphadenopathy

Diagnostic tests
■ *Laboratory tests:* check CBC, liver function tests, rapid plasma reagin (RPR), gonorrhea/chlamydia, Pap smear, purified protein derivative (PPD) testing to exclude tuberculosis
■ *Specific diagnostic tests:* check viral load; viral genotype/susceptibilities, if indicated
■ *Imaging tests:* ultrasound q 3–4 wk from 28 wk for fetal growth
■ *Screening tests:* offer HIV testing to all women at first prenatal visit; repeat later in pregnancy in women at high risk

DIFFERENTIAL DIAGNOSIS
■ Hepatitis B, C
■ Pneumonia
■ Anorexia

COMPLICATIONS
■ *Maternal complications:* increased risk of preterm premature rupture of membranes, preterm labor
■ *Fetal complications:* vertical transmission, prematurity

PROGNOSIS

■ Pregnancy does not increase progression to AIDS

MANAGEMENT

General measures

■ Check CBC, liver function tests q month
■ Check viral load q trimester if stable or 4–6 wk after change in Rx
■ Regular ID consultation

Specific treatment

■ Antiretroviral Rx in consultation w/ HIV specialist; compliance important; use multidrug regimen to prevent resistance, incl:
  ➤ Nucleocide inhibitors (AZT, DDI, 3TC, D4T)
  ➤ Protease inhibitors (indinavir, nelfinavir, ritonivir, sequanavir)
  ➤ Others (nivaripine, delacirone, etacirenz)
■ *Pneumocystis carinii* pneumonia prophylaxis, if indicated (CD4 <200)
■ Tuberculosis prophylaxis, if indicated (CD4 <50)
■ Amniocentesis relatively contraindicated given potential risk of transmission
  ➤ Discuss delivery; recommend elective cesarean at 38 wk (no amnio) for viral load >1,000 copies/mL
■ If vaginal delivery planned, avoid early amniotomy, prolonged rupture of membranes, fetal scalp electrode placement

Side effects & complications of treatment

■ Rash, bone marrow depression, liver dysfunction secondary to antiretroviral medications

SUBSEQUENT MANAGEMENT

■ Follow-up w/ HIV specialist

HYDROPS FETALIS

BACKGROUND

- Latin for "edema of fetus"
- Abnormal fluid accumulation in $>=2$ extravascular compartments (pleural/pericardial effusion, ascites, skin edema, placental edema)
- *Incidence:* <1% of pregnancies; 1/2,000 births
- *Classification / etiology:*
    1. *Nonimmune hydrops* (90%): due to cardiac (20–35%), chromosomal anomalies (15%), anemia (10%), other (infection, twin-twin transfusion syndrome); 50–60% no known cause
    2. *Immune hydrops* (10%): due to blood group incompatibility (ABO; D [Rh] rare)

DIAGNOSIS

History

- May have rapid increased abdominal girth, weight gain; decreased fetal activity

Physical examination

- Uterine size > dates (polyhydramnios in 50–75%)

Diagnostic tests

- Ultrasound Dx
- Look for cause: check type & screen, serologic screening (for toxoplasmosis, rubella, CMV, HSV), Hb electrophoresis, fetal karyotype, Kleihauer-Betke test (for fetomaternal hemorrhage), fetal anatomic survey, middle cerebral artery velocity to suggest fetal anemia

DIFFERENTIAL DIAGNOSIS

- Isolated polyhydramnios
- Abnormal fluid collection in 1 fetal body cavity

COMPLICATIONS

- *Maternal complications:* preterm premature rupture of membranes, preterm labor, preeclampsia/mirror syndrome
- *Fetal complications:* stillbirth, intrauterine growth restriction, prematurity

PROGNOSIS

- Depends on etiology, gestational age, severity of hydrops
- Overall prognosis poor w/ perinatal mortality rate >50% independent of gestational age

MANAGEMENT

General measures

- Confirm Dx, identify cause
- Timing, route of delivery depend on severity, gestational age
- Consider pregnancy termination

Specific treatment

- >32 wk, deliver (consider paracentesis, thoracocentesis to facilitate vaginal delivery, aid in resuscitation)
- Immune hydrops: serial antibody titers; amniotic fluid delta-OD450 at 22–32 wk, if indicated; results dictate future Mx (delivery, repeat delta-OD450, percutaneous umbilical cord sampling, transfusion)
- Recently, serial middle cerebral artery (MCA) Doppler for fetal anemia has replaced need for amnio and amniotic fluid delta-OD450
- Neonatology consult
- Consider antenatal corticosteroids
- Serial ultrasound to monitor progression, response to Rx

Prevention

- Can prevent Rh isoimmunization: RhoGAM (anti-D IgG) to Rh(−) women after abortion, ectopic, chorionic villus sampling, amniocentesis, bleeding, routinely at 28–32 wk, after delivery of Rh (+) fetus

Screening

■ Check antibody status at 1st prenatal visit

■ If mother isoimmunized, check father's blood group, antibody status

SUBSEQUENT MANAGEMENT

■ Recurrence rare for nonimmune, common for immune hydrops

HYPEREMESIS GRAVIDARUM (HEG)

BACKGROUND

■ NVP complicates 70–85% of all pregnancies; 1.3% have hyperemesis (unremitting severe NVP leading to dehydration, ketosis, weight loss)

■ Etiology unclear

■ First-trimester Dx; resolves on average by 17 wk; persists to term in 5–15%

■ Not limited to any socioeconomic, educational, age group

DIAGNOSIS

History

■ Ask about NVP (nausea and vomiting of pregnancy) in prior pregnancy

■ 1/3 have increased salivation (ptyalism)

■ *Trigger factors:* hyperolfaction (to perfume, chemicals, pets, food), heat & humidity (may concentrate odors & pollutants), noise, visual & physical motion (computer screen, elevators), prenatal supplements

Physical examination

■ Usually unhelpful

Diagnostic tests

- *Laboratory tests:* check ketones; serum electrolytes (albumin poor marker of nutrition in pregnancy)
- *Specific diagnostic tests:* none, clinical Dx

DIFFERENTIAL DIAGNOSIS

- Hyperthyroidism
- Primary psychiatric Dx
- Peptic ulcer disease

COMPLICATIONS

- *Maternal complications:* dehydration, weight loss, electrolyte abnormalities, malnutrition; rarely Wernicke's encephalopathy, splenic avulsion, aspiration, esophageal rupture
- *Fetal complications:* rare

PROGNOSIS

- HEG assoc. w/ improved pregnancy outcome

MANAGEMENT

General measures

- Intervene early
- Consider dietitian consult

Specific treatment

- Lifestyle changes (identify & minimize triggers, mask odors w/ lemon)
- Correct dehydration, electrolyte abnormalities
- Nutritional support (total parenteral nutrition; nasogastric, gastrostomy feeding)
- Dietary modifications: ginger, decreased fat intake, pyridoxine (vitamin B_6), ? vitamin B_1 (thiamine)
- *Pharmacologic treatment:*
  1. Antiemetics: metoclopramide, droperidol, odansetron
  2. Antihistamines: chlorpheniramine, doxylamine, diphenhydramine, trimethobenzamide, meclizine,

3. Phenothiazines/antipsychotics: prochlorperazine, chlorpromazine, promethazine
4. Other: methylprednisolone, adrenocorticotropic hormone
- Consider hospitalization if unresponsive
- Alternative Mx (acupressure, acupuncture, psychotherapy, hypnotherapy, homeopathy) of unclear benefit

Contraindications
- Bendectin (doxylamine + pyridoxine) effective; only FDA-approved drug for NVP; withdrawn from market in 1983 due to unfounded concerns about teratogenicity

SUBSEQUENT MANAGEMENT
- Increased recurrence rate in subsequent pregnancies

HYPERTHYROIDISM

BACKGROUND
- Circulating levothyroxine (T4) & L-triiodothyronine (T3) bound to thyroxine-binding globulin (TBG) w/ <1% as free (biologically active) hormone; iodine required for thyroid hormone production
- Pregnancy increases TBG leading to increases in total T4 & T3, but free T4, T3, & TSH levels remain unchanged
- <0.1% of thyroid hormone crosses placenta; tests of fetal thyroid function independent of maternal thyroid status but dependent on iodine from mother; thyroid hormone can be measured in fetal blood at 12 wk
- Maternal hyperthyroidism occurs in 0.05–0.2% of pregnancies

DIAGNOSIS
History
- May be asymptomatic

- Sx may be subtle, incl. emotional lability, anxiety, lethargy, fatigue, palpitations, heat intolerance, infertility, oligomenorrhea, diarrhea, weight loss, urinary frequency

Physical examination

- Signs may incl. tachycardia, hair loss, fine tremor, sweating, warm skin, ± thyromegaly (w/ or w/o bruit, dysphagia), proximal myopathy, pretibial myxedema; serious features incl. cardiac failure, dysrhythmias
- Eye signs (ophthalmopathy) such as exophthalmos specific to Graves' disease

Diagnostic tests

- Thyroid function tests (TFTs) required for definitive Dx; TSH most sensitive index of thyroid dysfunction in pregnancy
- Laboratory tests may show anemia, increased liver function tests, hypercalcemia, ± thyroid-stimulating antibodies (although none of these tests are diagnostic)

DIFFERENTIAL DIAGNOSIS

- Abnormal TFTs secondary to drug effect (iodine, glucocorticoids, sulfonylureas, cimetidine, phenytoin, lithium, dopamine agonists)
- Since hCG (human chorionic gonadotropin) is similar to TSH, conditions assoc. w/ increased hCG (hyperemesis gravidarum, gestational trophoblastic neoplasia) may show biochemical evidence of hyperthyroidism but rarely sx or signs
- Exogenous T4 or T3
- Struma ovarii (thyroid tissue in mature ovarian teratoma)
- Metastatic follicular cell carcinoma of thyroid (rare)

COMPLICATIONS

- *Maternal complications:* infertility, spontaneous abortion, cardiac failure (10–20%), thyroid storm (<0.1%)
- *Fetal complications:* preterm birth, intrauterine growth restriction, stillbirth

PROGNOSIS

- Graves' disease accounts for 95% of hyperthyroidism in pregnancy; thyroid-stimulating IgG can cross placenta, leading to fetal thyroid dysfunction; fetal tachycardia (>160 bpm) most sensitive measure of fetal hyperthyroidism

MANAGEMENT

General measures

- Goal: to control hyperthyroidism while avoiding fetal &/or transient neonatal hypothyroidism
- Antithyroid drugs Rx of choice; propylthiouracil (PTU), methimazole both effective; PTU preferred since methimazole assoc. w/ aplasia cutis congenita
- Radioactive iodine to ablate thyroid absolutely contraindicated in pregnancy
- Surgery best avoided in pregnancy but if indicated best performed in 2nd trimester

Specific treatment

- Check TFTs in pregnancy if clinical features suggest thyroid dysfunction; routine TSH screening of all pregnant women not recommended
- Initiate PTU (100–150 mg po tid) if indicated
- Check TSH levels q 4–6 wk & adjust PTU dose to keep TSH at 0.5–5 mU/L
- Check CBC q month (because of risk of PTU-induced agranulocytosis)
- Regular fetal testing (serial ultrasound for fetal growth, evidence of thyroid dysfunction incl. fetal goiter, fetal heart rate abnormalities; check weekly fetal heart rate after 32 wk)

SUBSEQUENT MANAGEMENT

- Check TFTs 6–8 wk after delivery
- Reconsider Mx as indicated

HYPOTHYROIDISM

BACKGROUND
- Circulating levothyroxine (T4) & L-triiodothyronine (T3) bound to thyroxine-binding globulin (TBG) w/ <1% as free (biologically active) hormone; iodine required for thyroid hormone production
- Pregnancy increases TBG, leading to increases in total T4 & T3, but free T4, T3, & TSH levels remain unchanged
- <0.1% of thyroid hormone crosses placenta; tests of fetal thyroid function independent of maternal thyroid status but dependent on iodine from mother; thyroid hormone can be measured in fetal blood at 12 wk
- Primary maternal hypothyroidism rare in pregnancy

DIAGNOSIS

History
- May be asymptomatic
- Sx may be subtle, incl. menorrhagia, infertility, weight gain, cold intolerance, lethargy, fatigue, constipation, depression, psychosis
- History of prior Rx (irradiation, surgery) for hyperthyroidism w/ or w/o thyroid hormone replacement

Physical examination
- Signs may incl. hair loss, hoarse voice, delayed tendon reflexes, brittle nails, coarse facial features (periorbital puffiness, expressionless face, large tongue) ± thyromegaly; serious features incl. pericardial effusion, cardiomyopathy
- Tender, swollen thyroid ± fever suggests suppurative (infectious) or subacute (viral) thyroiditis

Diagnostic tests
- Thyroid function tests (TFTs) required for definitive Dx; TSH most sensitive index of thyroid dysfunction in pregnancy

- Laboratory tests may show anemia, increased lactate dehydrogenase, increased cholesterol, increased creatine phosphokinase, ± antithyroid antibodies (none of these tests are diagnostic)

DIFFERENTIAL DIAGNOSIS
- Consider iodine deficiency (rare)
- Abnormal TFTs secondary to drug effect (iodine, glucocorticoids, propylthiouracil, sulfonylureas, cimetidine, phenytoin, lithium, dopamine agonists)
- Postpartum thyroiditis (transient hyperthyroid state 2–3 mo postpartum or transient hypothyroid state 4–8 mo postpartum; occurs in 4–10% of all postpartum women)

COMPLICATIONS
- *Maternal complications:* infertility, recurrent pregnancy loss, placental abruption, spontaneous abortion
- *Fetal complications:* stillbirth, intrauterine growth restriction, impaired neonatal & childhood development (cretinism)

PROGNOSIS
- Subclinical maternal hypothyroidism in pregnancy may be assoc. w/ long-term cognitive deficits in offspring but routine TSH screening of all pregnant women not recommended
- Women treated for Graves' disease may be asymptomatic but their fetuses remain at risk because of presence of circulating antithyroid IgG antibodies; check fetal heart rate on regular basis (fetal tachycardia most sensitive measure of fetal hyperthyroidism)

MANAGEMENT
General measures
- Confirm Dx
- If indicated, initiate levothyroxine (Synthroid) Rx at 100–150 mcg/d

- In women on Synthroid prior to conception, continue at prepregnancy dose

Specific treatment

- Check TFTs in pregnancy if clinical features suggest thyroid dysfunction; routine TSH screening of all pregnant women not recommended
- Check TSH levels q 4–6 wk & adjust Synthroid dose as indicated to keep TSH at 0.5–5 mU/L; most women need to increase dose by 30–50% in pregnancy
- Regular fetal testing (serial ultrasound examinations for fetal growth)
- Effect delivery by 39–40 wk if poorly controlled

SUBSEQUENT MANAGEMENT

- Postpartum thyroiditis may recur in subsequent pregnancy & progress to permanent hypothyroidism

---

IDIOPATHIC THROMBOCYTOPENIC PURPURA (ITP)

BACKGROUND

- Autoimmune disease characterized by circulating antiplatelet antibodies & maternal thrombocytopenia
- Incidence: 1–3/1,000 pregnancies

DIAGNOSIS

History

- Dx usually made prior to pregnancy
- Ask about easy bruising; excessive bleeding w/ surgery, dental procedures

Physical examination

- Usually unhelpful
- Check for splenomegaly, signs of thrombocytopenia (petechiae, subconjunctival hemorrhage, bleeding gums)

Diagnostic tests

- *Laboratory tests:* check platelet count
- *Specific diagnostic tests:* may check antiplatelet antibody titer (but correlates poorly w/ platelet count in either mother or fetus)
- *Imaging:* not routinely indicated
- *Screening:* routinely check platelet count at 1st prenatal visit & in 3rd trimester

DIFFERENTIAL DIAGNOSIS

- Gestational thrombocytopenia
- Preeclampsia
- DIC
- Drug-induced thrombocytopenia
- SLE
- Alloimmune thrombocytopenia (ATP) distinct from ITP, analogous to Rh disease of platelets; refers to antiplatelet antibodies (usually anti-PLA1) that cross placenta to cause fetal thrombocytopenia & possibly intraventricular hemorrhage; maternal platelet counts normal

COMPLICATIONS

- *Maternal complications:* excessive bleeding, complications of regional anesthesia (spinal hematoma)
- *Fetal complications:* rare (antiplatelet IgG can cross placenta & cause fetal thrombocytopenia, but correlation between maternal & fetal platelet count poor; antepartum intraventricular hemorrhage possible)

PROGNOSIS

- Majority of pregnancies uneventful

MANAGEMENT

General measures

- Follow maternal platelet counts q 3–4 wk

- Antepartum anesthesia consult
- Consider delivery >36 wk

Specific treatment
- Consider corticosteroids if maternal thrombocytopenia <70,000/mcL
- Splenectomy rarely indicated in pregnancy
- Regional anesthesia contraindicated if thrombocytopenia severe (<70,000/mcL)
- Mode of delivery: no proven benefit to elective cesarean (unless fetal platelet count <50,000/mcL by antepartum percutaneous umbilical blood sampling or intrapartum fetal scalp platelets, but neither procedure routinely recommended)

Contraindications
- Avoid operative vaginal delivery, unless fetal platelet count known to be >100,000/mcL
  - ➢ Avoid placement of fetal scalp electrode
- Breastfeeding not contraindicated

Side effects & complications of treatment
- Corticosteroids (prednisone) do not cross placenta to any great extent; as such, no known adverse fetal effects

SUBSEQUENT MANAGEMENT
- Hematology follow-up postpartum

INDUCTION OF LABOR

BACKGROUND
- Refers to interventions to initiate labor prior to spontaneous onset to achieve vaginal delivery

DIAGNOSIS

History
- Confirm gestational age, no contraindications to labor/ vaginal delivery

Physical examination
- Check fetal presentation, clinical estimated fetal weight, clinical pelvimetry, cervical exam

Diagnostic tests
- Check fetal lung maturity, sonographic estimated fetal weight, if indicated

DIFFERENTIAL DIAGNOSIS
- Different from augmentation, which refers to enhancement of uterine contractility in laboring women

COMPLICATIONS
- *Maternal complications:* failed induction leading to cesarean
- *Fetal complications:* rare

PROGNOSIS
- Success depends on cervical exam (Bishop score >=6, favorable; <6 assoc. w/ failed induction)

MANAGEMENT

General measures
- Induction recommended when risk/benefit equation favors delivery; gestational age-dependent
- Confirm indications:
  1. *Absolute:* maternal (preeclampsia, diabetes, renal/pulmonary disease), fetal (chorioamnionitis, isoimmunization, postterm, intrauterine growth restriction, abnormal fetal testing), uteroplacental (abruption)
  2. *Relative:* maternal (hypertension, gestational diabetes), fetal (intrauterine fetal demise, premature rupture of

membranes, prior intrauterine fetal demise, congenital anomaly), uteroplacental (oligohydramnios)

Specific treatment
- If cervix favorable, consider oxytocin, amniotomy (avoid in women w/ active herpes simplex virus, HIV)
- If cervix unfavorable, consider cervical ripening to decrease failed inductions, cesarean rate, maternal/fetal morbidity:
  1. *Effective:* PGE2 (dinoprostone gel [Prepidil], sustained release [Cervidil]; avoid in women w/ asthma, glaucoma, severe renal/pulmonary/hepatic disease); PGE1 (misoprostol [Cytotec]; not FDA approved); oxytocin; mechanical dilators
  2. *Ineffective:* stripping membranes
  3. *Investigational:* steroid receptor antagonists, relaxin

Side effects & complications of treatment
- Uterine hypertonus, tachysystole (prostaglandin [PG], oxytocin)
- Uterine rupture (esp. PG w/ prior cesarean)
- GI side effects (PG)
- Maternal water intoxication (oxytocin)

Contraindications to induction
- *Absolute:* maternal (active genital herpes), fetal (malpresentation, nonreassuring fetal testing), uteroplacental (cord prolapse, previa, vasa previa, prior classical cesarean, full-thickness myomectomy)
- Cytotec contraindicated in women w/ prior cesarean
- *Relative:* maternal (prior cesarean, cervical cancer, pelvic deformity), fetal (macrosomia), uteroplacental (marginal previa, bleeding)

SUBSEQUENT MANAGEMENT
- Depends on indication for & success of induction

INTRAPARTUM FETAL TESTING

BACKGROUND
- Fetal morbidity/mortality can occur as consequence of labor
- Dx of intrapartum fetal hypoxic ischemic encephalopathy (HIE) requires acidemia (pH <7.0), Apgar 0–3 for >5 min, neurologic sequelae, & multisystem organ failure; at most, 15% of cerebral palsy due to intrapartum HIE

DIAGNOSIS
History
- Check fetal movements

Physical examination
- Intermittent auscultation of fetal heart rate in labor as effective as electronic monitoring

DIFFERENTIAL DIAGNOSIS
- Many causes of cerebral injury (intraventricular hemorrhage, HIE, infection, trauma, metabolic disorders, drugs)

COMPLICATIONS
- *Maternal complications:* increased operative vaginal delivery, cesarean
- *Fetal complication:* HIE, death

PROGNOSIS
- Intrapartum testing increases obstetric intervention; unclear if improves perinatal outcome

MANAGEMENT
General measures
- Interpret tests in light of gestational age, congenital anomalies, clinical risk factors
- Able to perform emergent cesarean if necessary

Specific diagnostic tests

1. *Electronic fetal heart rate monitoring:* check baseline (110–160 bpm), variability (peak-to-trough 6–25 bpm), accelerations (>=15 bpm x >=15 sec if >=32 wk; >=10 bpm x >=10 sec if <32 wk), decelerations (early, variable, late; periodic or episodic; prolonged, recurrent); interpretation is subjective (1997 NICHHD guidelines):
   - ➤ *Reassuring* (normal baseline & variability, accelerations & no decelerations)
   - ➤ *At risk* (recurrent late or variable decelerations w/ absent variability; prolonged bradycardia); seen in 0.3% of labors; associated w/ adverse outcome in 35–40% of cases; consider immediate delivery
   - ➤ *Intermediate* (any other pattern); seen in 60% of labors
2. *Scalp stimulation:* acceleration predicts pH >7.20
3. *Fetal scalp sampling:* pH of fetal capillary blood between arterial & venous; suggested Mx:
   - ➤ pH >7.25: confirms fetal well-being
   - ➤ pH 7.20–7.25: repeat q 20–30 min
   - ➤ pH <7.20: immediate delivery
4. *Other:* biophysical profile (poorly validated in labor), fetal pulse oximetry (investigational)

Contraindications to labor

■ Previa, nonreassuring fetal testing, prior high vertical hysterotomy/full-thickness myomectomy, prior uterine rupture, transverse lie, ? breech

SUBSEQUENT MANAGEMENT

■ Specific to suspected pathology

INTRAUTERINE FETAL DEMISE

BACKGROUND

■ IUFD (stillbirth) refers to fetal demise prior to delivery
■ Overall stillbirth rate in U.S.: 7.5–9/1,000 births

DIAGNOSIS

History

■ Suspect Dx if sx of normal pregnancy subside (nausea, frequency, breast tenderness)

■ In later pregnancy, suspect Dx if fetal movements absent or decreased

■ *Risk factors:* extremes of maternal age, multiple pregnancy, postterm pregnancy, macrosomia, fetal anomalies, cocaine, smoking, maternal disease (diabetes, thyroid disease, hypertension), abnormal placentation (placenta previa, abruption)

Physical examination

■ Suspect Dx if no uterine growth or no fetal heart rate tones audible

Diagnostic tests

■ *Imaging tests:* ultrasound shows absence of fetal cardiac activity; scalp edema, fetal maceration may be evident

■ Abdominal x-ray signs (overlapping of skull bones [Spalding sign], gas in fetus, excessive curvature of fetal spine) of historical interest only

DIFFERENTIAL DIAGNOSIS

■ None

COMPLICATIONS

■ *Maternal complication:* DIC occurs in 20–25% if nonviable singleton fetus is retained for >=3 wk (does not occur following IUFD of 1 twin)

■ *Fetal complications:* IUFD of 1 dizygous twin rarely affects its cotwin (because they do not share circulation); IUFD of 1 monozygous twin may rarely lead to IUFD of its cotwin (<2%) but often (15–25%) leads to irreversible neurologic injury (multicystic encephalomalacia)

PROGNOSIS

- Latency (period from IUFD to delivery) depends on underlying cause & gestational age; most women deliver w/in 1–2 wk
- Prognosis for surviving cotwin depends on gestational age, cause of death, & chorionicity

MANAGEMENT

General measures

- Every effort should be made to avoid cesarean delivery
- Parents should be allowed to grieve (encouraged to hold their lost child; to name him/her)

Specific treatment

- For singleton IUFD, expectant Mx may be recommended for 1–2 wk; thereafter, D&C or induction of labor
- Individualization of Mx important (some parents find idea of going home w/ nonviable pregnancy overwhelming & request immediate delivery)
- Mx of surviving cotwin depends on chorionicity & gestational age; fetal well-being should be assessed on regular basis (weekly) & delivery effected once fetal lung maturity confirmed or favorable gestational age reached

Contraindications

- DIC, nonreassuring fetal testing in surviving cotwin are contraindications to expectant Mx

SUBSEQUENT MANAGEMENT

- Recurrence rate depends on cause
- Following delivery, make every effort to find cause of IUFD: fetopsy incl. pathologic examination of placenta is single most useful investigation; Kleihauer-Betke test (to document significant fetomaternal hemorrhage); infection (can culture

placenta, uterus); fetal karyotype; antiphospholipid antibody syndrome
- >50% of cases have no known cause

INTRAUTERINE GROWTH RESTRICTION (IUGR)

BACKGROUND
- Refers to any fetus that fails to achieve full growth potential
- Birthweight: function of growth rate (dependent on genetic factors, intrauterine environment) & gestational age
- Incidence: 4–8% of pregnancies in U.S.
- Distinction between asymmetric, symmetric IUGR not always clinically useful

DIAGNOSIS
History
- Often unhelpful
- *Risk factors:* prior IUGR, hypertension, vaginal bleeding, fetal anomalies, multiple gestations, fetal infections, tobacco/alcohol/cocaine abuse

Physical examination
- Uterine size < dates (but clinical Dx of IUGR unreliable)

Diagnostic tests
- *Laboratory tests:* unhelpful
- *Specific diagnostic tests:* check ultrasound for estimated fetal weight (EFW), structural anomalies, Doppler; karyotype
- *Imaging tests:* IUGR ultrasound Dx w/ EFW <10th percentile plus evidence of fetal compromise, ponderal index <10th percentile
- *Screening:* check fundal height

DIFFERENTIAL DIAGNOSIS
- Fetal aneuploidy
- Congenital anomaly of CNS, heart (except transposition, tetralogy)
- Infection (malaria, rubella, cytomegalovirus, toxoplasmosis, syphilis)
- Single umbilical artery, abnormal cord insertion
- Multiple gestation
- Uteroplacental insufficiency due to preeclampsia, thrombosis, abruption (*Note:* previa does not cause IUGR)
- Toxins (tobacco, alcohol, cocaine)

COMPLICATIONS
- *Maternal complications:* increased cesarean
- *Fetal complications:* prematurity, increased intrapartum nonreassuring fetal testing (25–50%), hypoglycemia, polycythemia, meconium aspiration syndrome, cerebral palsy

PROGNOSIS
- Morbidity increased w/ EFW <10th percentile; mortality increased w/ EFW <6th percentile

MANAGEMENT
General measures
- Identify pregnancies at high risk
- Early antepartum Dx
- Determine etiology, Rx underlying causes
- Consider delivery at favorable gestational age, once lung maturity confirmed or if abnormal fetal testing

Specific treatment
- Regular (twice weekly) fetal testing
  1. Nonstress test
  2. Biophysical profile (consider delivery for <4/10 or 6/10 if oligohydramnios)

3. Umbilical artery Doppler velocimetry (consider delivery for absent, reverse diastolic flow)
4. Contraction stress test
■ Neonatal consult & corticosteroid Rx if indicated

Prevention
■ Benefit of bedrest, acetylsalicylic acid in women at high risk unclear

SUBSEQUENT MANAGEMENT
■ Rx underlying causes of IUGR prior to subsequent pregnancy

ISOIMMUNIZATION

BACKGROUND
■ Refers to maternal sensitization to foreign blood group antigens
■ Differences in antigenicity lead to differences in fetal effects
■ Blood grp: ABO
  ➤ Disease?: ±
  ➤ Antigen: ABO
■ Blood grp: Rh
  ➤ Disease?: +++
  ➤ Antigen: D,C,c,E,e
■ Blood grp: Lewis
  ➤ Disease?: –
  ➤ Antigen: Le[a/b]
■ Blood grp: Kell
  ➤ Disease?: +++
  ➤ Antigen: K,k,Js,Kp
■ Blood grp: Kidd
  ➤ Disease?: +
  ➤ Antigen: Jk[a/b],Jk3

- Blood grp: Duffy
  - ➤ Disease?: ++
  - ➤ Antigen: Fy[a,b],Fy3
- Blood grp: Lutheran
  - ➤ Disease?: +
  - ➤ Antigen: Lu[a/b]

DIAGNOSIS

History
- Ask about prior hemolytic disease, maternal blood transfusion
- Decreased fetal movement

Physical examination
- Serial BP, weight, fundal height

Diagnostic tests
- *Laboratory tests:* check paternal antigen status
- *Specific diagnostic tests:* serial maternal antibody titers at 1st visit, 20 wk, then q 3–4 wk: <=1:8, no action; >=1:16 (albumin) or >=1:32 (Coombs), further action required
- *Imaging tests:* serial ultrasound for fetal hydrops (develops when HCT <15%)
- *Screening tests:* check antibody titers in all parturients at 1st prenatal visit & in 3rd trimester; middle cerebral artery (MCA) Doppler velocimetry, delta-OD450 (largely supplanted by MCA velocimetry), & occasionally percutaneous umbilical blood sampling for fetal HCT (see Mx)

DIFFERENTIAL DIAGNOSIS
- Nonimmune hydrops (incl. fetal infection, genetic disorders, fetal hemorrhage, metabolic disease, cardiac anomalies/arrhythmias)

COMPLICATIONS
- *Fetal complications:* increased intrauterine fetal demise related to severity of disease or Rx (percutaneous umbilical blood sampling ~1%, intrauterine transfusion [IUT] 4–9%)

■ *Maternal complications:* rarely preeclampsia-like "mirror" syndrome

PROGNOSIS
■ Correlates w/ delta-OD450 (except Kell): Liley Zone I: good prognosis; Zone II: may need IUT; Zone III: poor prognosis (>90% risk of intrauterine fetal demise in 1 wk): consider IUT, delivery
■ Perinatal survival rates >80% w/ IUT

MANAGEMENT

General measures
■ Amniocentesis for fetal antigen status if father heterozygous
■ Amniocentesis for optical density (delta-OD450), which reflects bilirubin content of fluid & is indirect measure of hemolysis; now largely replaced by MCA Doppler
■ Serial MCA Doppler velocimetry for fetal anemia

Specific treatment
■ IUT, if indicated; repeat as needed to keep HCT 20–25% (allow 1%/d decrease in HCT)
■ Immediate delivery if severely affected & >=32 wk

Contraindications
■ To IUT: maternal anticoagulation, >32 wk, minimal fetal disease

Side effects & complications of treatment
■ Preterm premature rupture of membranes, iatrogenic prematurity
■ Intrauterine fetal demise
■ Fetal hemorrhage

Follow-up care
■ Zone I: reassess q3–4 wk, deliver at term
■ Zone II: reassess q1–4 wk, deliver 36–38 wk

■ Zone III: immediate intervention (IUT <32 wk; delivery vs. IUT >=32 wk)

SUBSEQUENT MANAGEMENT
■ Successive affected pregnancies w/ same father more severely affected

---

LISTERIA

BACKGROUND
■ Refers to infection w/ *Listeria monocytogenes*, an anaerobic, Gram-positive rod that produces beta-hemolysis on blood agar
■ Rare in population at large but increases 20-fold in pregnancy
■ Pathogenesis poorly understood; epidemics have been assoc. w/ ingestion of contaminated food, esp. nonpasteurized dairy products
■ Vertical transmission occurs most likely by hematogenous dissemination at time of maternal septicemia

DIAGNOSIS
History
■ Dx requires high index of suspicion
■ May give Hx (in retrospect) of ingestion of nonpasteurized dairy products

Physical examination
■ 2/3 of pregnant women present w/ fever, headache, myalgias, & other nonspecific flu-like symptoms; 1/3 experience primarily GI sx (diarrhea)
■ Severe complications (encephalitis, meningitis, ARDS, death) usually assoc. w/ underlying immunosuppression
■ Maternal fever, preterm labor (esp. in setting of nonreassuring fetal testing), & unexplained intrauterine fetal demise

raise possibility of acute listeriosis, even in absence of clinical chorioamnionitis

Diagnostic tests

- Dx confirmed by isolation of *L. monocytogenes* from maternal or neonatal blood, fetal membranes, gastric aspirates, amniotic fluid, or placental tissues
- Amniotic fluid infected w/ *Listeria* is characteristic light-green color
- Histologic evidence of multifocal villitis, microabscesses in placenta can confirm Dx following delivery
- Consider sending nonpasteurized dairy products to state lab for analysis

DIFFERENTIAL DIAGNOSIS

- Other causes of fetal infection, preterm labor
- Light-green amniotic fluid can be confused w/ meconium

COMPLICATIONS

- *Maternal complications:* abortion, chorioamnionitis, preterm labor
- *Fetal complications:* intrauterine fetal demise/neonatal death, preterm birth, sepsis

PROGNOSIS

- Adverse pregnancy outcome can occur at any gestational age
- Accounts for estimated 1–3% of abortion & preterm delivery
- Overall perinatal mortality ranges from 20–50%

MANAGEMENT

General measures

- If *Listeria* infection suspected, prompt IV antibiotics may improve perinatal outcome
- Perinatal outcome determined primarily by gestational age at delivery & complications related to prematurity

Specific treatment
- Confirm Dx
- Document fetal well-being
- Clinical trials have yet to identify most appropriate Rx; commonly used regimens incl. IV ampicillin/gentamicin or IV trimethoprim/sulfamethoxazole & erythromycin
- Proceed w/ immediate delivery if gestational age favorable or if evidence of fetal compromise
- Neonates should receive IV broad-spectrum antibiotics, although length of therapy is unknown

Prevention
- Avoid all nonpasteurized foods in pregnancy, esp. dairy products such as soft cheese
- Currently no vaccine

SUBSEQUENT MANAGEMENT
- *Listeria* can recur if infected foods are reingested

LYME DISEASE

BACKGROUND
- Infection caused by spirochete, *Borrelia burgdorferi* (*B. garinii*, *B. afzelii* in Europe)
- Transmitted by bite of deer tick (*Ixodes dammini*, *I. scapularis*) or western black-legged tick (*I. pacificus*)
- Most common vector-borne disease in U.S. (12,500 cases/y)

DIAGNOSIS

History
- Hx of tick exposure or hiking in tick-infected areas w/in 30 d (Hx of tick bite not required for Dx); May-August is high risk in northern hemisphere
- Risk of Lyme disease after tick bite estimated at <5%

- Incubation period of 7–14 d followed by nonspecific flu-like sx (fever, malaise, fatigue, headache, myalgias, polyarthralgias) & characteristic rash
- Some infected individuals asymptomatic or experience only mild sx in early stage disease

Physical examination
- May be unhelpful
- Characteristic "bull's-eye" rash (erythema migrans) at site of tick bite in 60–80% of patients; lesions fade in 3–4 wk even w/o Rx
- Manifestations of late disease (4–6 wk after infection) incl. cranial nerve palsies, meningitis, myositis, asymmetric arthritis

Diagnostic tests
- Serologic tests of variable sensitivity & specificity; CDC recommends initial screening w/ enzyme-linked immunosorbent assay (ELISA) or indirect fluorescent antibody test (Western immunoblot used only when results equivocal)

DIFFERENTIAL DIAGNOSIS
- Other tick-borne infections (Rocky Mountain spotted fever, tularemia, ehrlichiosis)
- Disseminated gonococcal infection
- SLE

COMPLICATIONS
- *Maternal complications:* heart block, pericarditis, cardiomyopathy, motor & sensory peripheral neuropathy, meningitis, encephalitis, cranial nerve palsies, hepatitis, iritis, skin lesions (acrodermatitis chronica atrophicans)
- *Fetal complications:* stillbirth, preterm birth, long-term neurologic sequelae, delayed neonatal effects (SIDS)
- Lyme disease not teratogenic

PROGNOSIS

■ *B. burgdorferi* can infect placenta & fetus, but precise risk to fetus at various gestational ages not known

■ Overall risk of adverse pregnancy outcome appears low

■ Anti-*Borrelia* IgG persists for months or years but does not confer lifelong immunity from reinfection

MANAGEMENT

General measures

■ Aggressive Rx recommended to decrease fetal/neonatal infection but efficacy of this approach unclear

■ Rx if clinical suspicion high or once Dx confirmed

■ Early & aggressive antibiotic Rx may blunt antibody response, making Dx hard to confirm

Specific treatment

■ Doxycycline Rx of choice but contraindicated in pregnancy

■ In pregnancy, Rx w/ amoxicillin po for 3–4 wk; alternative Rx incl. cefuroxime, erythromycin

■ IV ceftriaxone or penicillin >=4 wk for advanced disease (esp. neurologic manifestations)

■ Rx failures do occur & some sx may persist even w/ successful treatment

Prevention

■ Prevent tick bites (avoid wooded areas, wear long pants, tick repellent)

■ Transmission takes place after >=2 d of feeding; identification & removal of ticks w/in 24 h effectively prevents transmission

■ Vaccine (LYMErix) to prevent Lyme disease does not protect all recipients against infection w/ *B. burgdorferi* & offers no protection against other tick-borne diseases; vaccination not recommended in pregnancy

SUBSEQUENT MANAGEMENT
- Prior infection or vaccination does not offer lifelong protection against reinfection w/ *B. burgdorferi* or other tick-borne disease
- Consider vaccination if living in high-risk area

MACROSOMIA

BACKGROUND
- Defined by ACOG as estimated fetal weight (not birth weight) >4,500 g; large-for-gestational age (LGA) refers to estimated fetal weight >90th percentile for gestational age
- In U.S., 5% of infants have birth weight >4,000 g & 0.5% have birth weight >4,500 g

DIAGNOSIS

History
- Usually asymptomatic
- In multipara, maternal estimation of fetal weight as accurate as clinical estimate by physician or ultrasound
- *Risk factors:* diabetes (major risk factor), postterm pregnancy, obesity, prior macrosomic infant, multiparity, male fetus, advancing maternal age, Beckwith-Wiedemann syndrome (pancreatic islet-cell hyperplasia); most women w/ risk factors have normal-weight babies

Physical examination
- Clinical estimates of fetal weight by Leopold maneuvers, fundal height measurements unreliable

Diagnostic tests
- Ultrasound can be used to estimate fetal weight based on measurements of abdominal circumference, femur length, & biparietal diameter; ultrasound estimation of fetal weight

± 20% of actual fetal weight (error may be greater in obese women)

DIFFERENTIAL DIAGNOSIS
- Incorrect dates
- Multiple pregnancy
- Obesity
- Uterine enlargement (fibroids, polyhydramnios)

COMPLICATIONS
- *Maternal complications:* increased cesarean delivery, post-partum hemorrhage, puerperal infection, perineal or vaginal trauma
- *Fetal complications:* increased risk of intrauterine fetal distress & neonatal death, birth trauma (brachial plexus injury); increased neonatal hypoglycemia, polycythemia, hypocalcemia, jaundice

PROGNOSIS
- Increased birth weight assoc. w/ increased risk of birth trauma, cesarean delivery, & maternal perineal injury
- Major risk to fetus: shoulder dystocia & resultant brachial plexus injury; most deliveries complicated by shoulder dystocia occur in fetuses weighing <4,000 g

MANAGEMENT
General measures
- Routine screening of all women for gestational diabetes at 24–28 wk; consider early screening (18–20 wk) in women at increased risk (prior gestational diabetes, prior macrosomic infant, obesity, family Hx of diabetes, sustained glycosuria)
- Meticulous glucose control in women w/ diabetes
- Because of association between macrosomia & cesarean delivery, early induction of labor for "impending macrosomia"

often considered; however, this approach has been shown not to decrease cesarean delivery rate & is not recommended

Specific treatment

■ Serial ultrasound examinations q 4–6 wk for fetal growth in pregnancies at risk for macrosomia

■ Check estimated fetal weight at 37–38 wk; consider recommending elective cesarean delivery for diabetic women w/ estimated fetal weight >4,500 g & for nondiabetic women w/ estimated fetal weight >5,000 g (because of increased risk of birth trauma)

■ Vaginal delivery of suspected macrosomic fetus should take place in controlled fashion, w/ access to obstetric anesthesia staff & neonatal resuscitation team; coordination between practitioner and supporting obstetric staff key to optimal management of shoulder dystocia; it is prudent to avoid assisted vaginal delivery in this setting

Prevention

■ Techniques to decrease fetal macrosomia include strict control of diabetes, prepregnancy weight loss &/or limited weight gain (only 20–25 lb) in obese pregnant women

SUBSEQUENT MANAGEMENT

■ Fetal macrosomia tends to recur in subsequent pregnancies

■ Women w/ gestational diabetes should be screened for type II diabetes 6–8 wk after delivery

MASTITIS

BACKGROUND

■ Incidence: 1–2% of lactating women

■ Can occur at any time while breastfeeding but occurs most commonly 10 d to 6 wk postpartum

- Typical organisms: *Staphyloccocus aureus, Haemophilus parainfluenzae, Escherichia coli*

DIAGNOSIS

History
- Unilateral breast pain, firmness
- May include fever, chills, malaise

Physical examination
- Check temperature
- Breast examination for segmental erythema, tenderness, firmness

Diagnostic tests
- *Laboratory tests:* check CBC & WBC differential
- *Specific diagnostic tests:* none; mastitis clinical Dx based on history, exam, & high index of clinical suspicion
- *Imaging tests:* consider breast ultrasound to exclude abscess
- *Screening tests:* patients should be told to call provider for postpartum fever or breast pain

DIFFERENTIAL DIAGNOSIS
- Obstructed milk duct
- Excessive engorgement
- Inflammatory breast carcinoma

COMPLICATIONS
- *Maternal complications:* breast abscess (esp. if *S. aureus*)
- *Fetal complications:* none

PROGNOSIS
- Early Dx & Rx highly successful at achieving cure
- Delay in Rx increases risk of abscess formation

MANAGEMENT

General measures
- Maintain adequate hydration while breastfeeding

- Continue breastfeeding or pumping throughout Rx
- Bedrest, as indicated
- Acetaminophen for fever, as needed

Specific treatment
- Repetitive manual expression of obstructed milk ducts
- Topical antibiotic Rx inadequate
- Appropriate Rx: dicloxacillin 500 mg po qid × 7–14 d; if penicillin-allergic, erythromycin 500 mg po bid × 7–14 d
- Surgical drainage of breast abscess

Contraindications
- Known allergies to above agents

Side effects & complications of treatment
- Increased risk of recurrence if Rx inadequate

Follow-up care
- Repeat breast exam after Rx

SUBSEQUENT MANAGEMENT
- Consider further evaluation (repeat breast ultrasound, surgical consult, mammography) to exclude breast carcinoma if mastitis fails to respond to Rx, recurs repeatedly, if palpable mass persists, or for bloody nipple discharge

---

MATERNAL ANEMIA

BACKGROUND
- Hemodilution of pregnancy causes 5% (2 g/dL) decreased HCT
- *Incidence:* 20–60% of parturients have HCT <35% in pregnancy
- *Causes:* (1) decreased red blood cell production (decreased reticulocytes); iron deficiency (microcytic, hypochromic

anemia), folate deficiency (megaloblastic anemia); (2) increased destruction: blood loss, sickle cell disease, thalassemia

DIAGNOSIS

History

- Asymptomatic or nonspecific sx (fatigue, dizziness, exertional dyspnea), rectal bleeding (change in character of stools)
- History of inflammatory bowel disease
- *Risk factors:* poor socioeconomic status; Mediterranean, Asian, African ancestry

Physical examination

- Pale mucous membranes, conjunctivae

Diagnostic tests

- *Laboratory tests:* Check HCT, hemoglobin
- *Specific diagnostic tests:*
  - ➤ MCV (macrocytic [MCV >100 fl] suggests folate, B_{12} deficiency; microcytic [MCV <80 fl] suggests iron deficiency, thalassemia)
  - ➤ Blood smear (hypersegmented neutrophils suggest megaloblastic or iron-deficiency anemia; hypochromic cells in iron deficiency; target cells & mean corpuscular hemoglobin <22 pg in thalassemia; malarial parasites)
    - Consider hemoglobin electrophoresis
  - ➤ Serum ferritin <35 mcg/L suggests iron deficiency (serum folate levels unreliable in pregnancy)
  - ➤ Consider consultation w/ a hematologist and possible bone marrow aspiration if anemia severe, Dx unclear
  - ➤ Check for intestinal parasites (esp. if recent immigrant, travel)
- *Imaging tests:* not routinely indicated
- *Screening tests:* routinely check CBC in 1st & 3rd trimesters, hemoglobin electrophoresis for hemoglobinopathies in select ethnic groups (not for alpha-thalassemia)

DIFFERENTIAL DIAGNOSIS
- Pancytopenia (myeloproliferative disorders, malaria)
- Intestinal parasites
- Drug-induced (eg, AZT causes macrocytic anemia)

COMPLICATIONS
- *Maternal complications:* blood transfusion; poor wound healing
- *Fetal complications:* intrauterine growth restriction (rare)

PROGNOSIS
- Depends on etiology, severity

MANAGEMENT
General measures
- Dietary consultation, encourage more consumption of red meat
- Offer genetic counseling in women w/ hemoglobinopathies

Specific treatment
- Iron Rx (ferrous sulfate 300 mg po qd, ferrous gluconate 320 mg po qd, ferrous fumarate 200 mg po qd)
- Folic acid 500 mcg po qd

Contraindications
- Limited role for IV iron or erythropoietin except in extreme cases (eg, Jehovah's Witness with placenta previa)

Side effects & complications of treatment
- Gastrointestinal upset, constipation w/ iron

Follow-up care
- Recheck HCT in 4 wk
- If anemia severe, check reticulocyte count & HCT in 2–5 d

SUBSEQUENT MANAGEMENT
- Hematology follow-up if indicated

MATERNAL CARDIAC DISEASE

BACKGROUND
- Accounts for 8% of maternal mortality in U.S. each year
- Complicates 1% of pregnancies

DIAGNOSIS

History
- Sx range from none to chest pain, dyspnea, orthopnea, edema, hemoptysis, palpitations
- Hx of congenital heart disease

Physical examination
- BP, detailed cardiac examination
- Assess hemodynamic stability

Diagnostic tests
- Cardiology consult, ECG, cardiac echocardiography
- Look for underlying cause, such as congenital heart lesions (>50%), thyroid dysfunction, hypertension, syphilis; rare causes include cardiac dysrhythmia, myocarditis/pericarditis, cardiomyopathy, coronary artery disease, rheumatic fever

Differential Diagnosis
- Pulmonary disease (interstitial lung disease, pneumonia, pulmonary edema, asthma)
- Pulmonary embolism
- Costochondritis
- Preeclampsia

COMPLICATIONS
- Depend on nature & severity of cardiac lesion
- *Maternal complications:* cardiac dysrhythmia, cardiac failure, cardiomyopathy, aortic dissection/rupture, preterm labor, maternal death

■ *Fetal complications:* prematurity, intrauterine growth restriction, stillbirth

PROGNOSIS

■ Prognosis variable; outcome influenced by several factors:

1. *Cardiac function:* New York Heart Association (NYHA) clinical classification: class I (no limitation of physical activity), class II (slight limitation), class III (symptoms w/ normal activity), class IV (sx at rest)
2. Coexisting medical conditions that may increase cardiac output (multiple pregnancy, anemia, thyroid disease)
3. *Medications*
4. Specific nature of *cardiac lesion*, classified into GROUP 1, mortality <1% (VSD, atrial septal defect, tetralogy of Fallot [surgically corrected], patent ductus arteriosus, pulmonary/tricuspid valve disease, bioprosthetic valve, mitral stenosis [NYHA class I, II]); GROUP 2, mortality 5–10% (2A: aortic stenosis, mitral stenosis [NYHA class III, IV], coarctation of aorta w/o valvular involvement, tetralogy of Fallot [uncorrected]) (2B: previous myocardial infarction, Marfan syndrome w/ normal aorta, mitral stenosis w/ atrial fibrillation, artificial valve); GROUP 3, mortality 25–50% (pulmonary hypertension, coarctation of aorta w/ valvular involvement, Marfan syndrome w/ aortic involvement)

MANAGEMENT

General measures

■ Regular prenatal care, assessment of sx, control BP
■ Cardiology consult, maternal echocardiography as indicated
■ Anticoagulation, if indicated
■ Anesthesia consult in late pregnancy
■ Fetal echocardiography at 18–22 wk in women w/ congenital heart disease to exclude fetal cardiac anomaly
■ Regular fetal testing (serial ultrasound exams for fetal growth)

- Timing & route of delivery depend on gestational age, condition of fetus & mother
- Cesarean delivery should be reserved for standard obstetric indications

Specific treatment

- Allow spontaneous labor at term; consider induction of labor in women requiring intrapartum invasive cardiac monitoring
- In labor, consider continuous pulse oximetry & ECG monitoring, strict intake & output monitoring (in women w/ fixed output cardiac lesions, avoid fluid overload)
- Supplemental oxygen & adequate pain relief (regional analgesia is preferred), as necessary
- Consider intrapartum invasive hemodynamic monitoring for women w/ NYHA class III & IV disease
- Consider elective shortening of 2nd stage of labor
- Autotransfusion of ~500 mL blood in immediate postpartum period may lead to hemodynamic compromise

SUBSEQUENT MANAGEMENT

- Congenital cardiac lesions inherited in multifactorial fashion; infants of women w/ congenital heart disease have 3–4% risk of inherited congenital cardiac disease
- Postpartum cardiomyopathy tends to recur in subsequent pregnancies

---

MATERNAL LABORATORY VALUES

TABLES

- Normal laboratory values are often different in pregnancy compared w/ nonpregnant state due to metabolic, physiologic, endocrine demands of pregnancy

HEMATOLOGIC TESTS

HCT (%)

- Nonpregnant: 37–47
- Pregnant: 33–44

Hgb (g/dL)

- Nonpregnant: 12–16
- Pregnant: 11–14

WBC (k/mm^3)

- Nonpregnant: 4.5–11
- Pregnant: 6–16

Platelets (k/mm^3)

- Nonpregnant: 130–400
- Pregnant: 120–350

Fibrinogen (ng/dL)

- Nonpregnant: 200–450
- Pregnant: 400–650

Ferritin (ng/mL)

- Nonpregnant: 25–120
- Pregnant: 15–150

Fe^{++} (mcg/dL)

- Nonpregnant: 135
- Pregnant: 90

TIBC (mcg/dL)

- Nonpregnant: 250–460
- Pregnant: 300–600

PT (sec)

- Nonpregnant: 12–14
- Pregnant: unchanged

PTT (sec)

- Nonpregnant: 24–36
- Pregnant: unchanged

Thrombin time (sec)

- Nonpregnant: 12–18
- Pregnant: unchanged

Factor VIII (%)

- Nonpregnant: 60–100
- Pregnant: 120–200

Factor X (%)

■ Nonpregnant: 60–100

■ Pregnant: 90–120

Factor IX (%)

■ Nonpregnant: 60–100

■ Pregnant: 90–120

Factors II,V,VII (%)

■ Nonpregnant: 60–100

■ Pregnant: unchanged

Factors XI,XIII (%)

■ Nonpregnant: 60–100

■ Pregnant: 40–60

SERUM CHEMISTRY

Na^+ (mEq/L)

■ Nonpregnant: 136–145

■ Pregnant: 130–140

K^+ (mEq/L)

■ Nonpregnant: 3.5–5.0

■ Pregnant: 3.3–4.1

HCO_3 (mEq/L)

■ Nonpregnant: 21–30

■ Pregnant: 18–25

Cl^- (mEq/L)

■ Nonpregnant: 98–106

■ Pregnant: 93–100

Cr (mg/dL)

■ Nonpregnant: <1.5

■ Pregnant: <0.8

BUN (mg/dL)

■ Nonpregnant: 10–20

■ Pregnant: 5–12

Mg^{++} (mg/dL)

■ Nonpregnant: 2–3

- Pregnant: 1.6–2.1

Total Ca^{++} (mg/dL)
- Nonpregnant: 9–10.5
- Pregnant: 8.1–9.5

Ion. Ca^{++} (mg/dL)
- Nonpregnant: 4.5–5.6
- Pregnant: 4–5

Uric acid (mg/dL)
- Nonpregnant: 1.5–6
- Pregnant: 1.2–4.5

Copper (ng/dL)
- Nonpregnant: 70–140
- Pregnant: 120–200

Phosphorus (mg/dL)
- Nonpregnant: 3–4.5
- Pregnant: unchanged

URINE CHEMISTRY

Protein (mg/24 h)
- Nonpregnant: <150
- Pregnant: <300

C. clear (mL/min)
- Nonpregnant: 91–130
- Pregnant: 120–160

ENDOCRINE TESTS

Fasting glu (mg/dL)
- Nonpregnant: 75–115
- Pregnant: 60–105

ACTH (pg/mL)
- Nonpregnant: 20–100
- Pregnant: unchanged

PTH (pg/mL)
- Nonpregnant: 20–30
- Pregnant: 10–20

Prolactin (ng/mL)
- Nonpregnant: 2–15
- Pregnant: 50–400

TSH (mcg/dL)
- Nonpregnant: 4–5
- Pregnant: unchanged

Total T4 (mcg/dL)
- Nonpregnant: 5–12
- Pregnant: 10–17

Free T4 (ng/dL)
- Nonpregnant: 1–2
- Pregnant: unchanged

T3 (ng/dL)
- Nonpregnant: 70–190
- Pregnant: 100–220

T3 resin uptake (%)
- Nonpregnant: 25–35
- Pregnant: 15–25

HEPATIC FUNCTION TESTS

Total bilirubin (mg/dL)
- Nonpregnant: 0.3–1
- Pregnant: unchanged

Total chol (mg/dL)
- Nonpregnant: 120–180
- Pregnant: 180–280

Triglyceride (mg/dL)
- Nonpregnant: <160
- Pregnant: <260

ALT (SGPT) (U/L)
- Nonpregnant: 0–35
- Pregnant: unchanged

AST (SGOT) (U/L)
- Nonpregnant: 0–35
- Pregnant: unchanged

PANCREATIC FUNCTION

Amylase (U/L)
- Nonpregnant: 60–180
- Pregnant: 90–350

Lipase (IU/dL)
- Nonpregnant: 4–24
- Pregnant: 2–12

OTHER TESTS

LDH (U/L)
- Nonpregnant: 200–450
- Pregnant: unchanged

CPK (U/L)
- Nonpregnant: 10–70
- Pregnant: 5–40

Albumin (g/dL)
- Nonpregnant: 3.5–5.5
- Pregnant: 2.5–4.5

IgG (mg/dL)
- Nonpregnant: 800–1500
- Pregnant: 700–1400

IgA (mg/dL)
- Nonpregnant: 90–325
- Pregnant: unchanged

IgM (mg/dL)
- Nonpregnant: 45–150
- Pregnant: unchanged

MULTIPLE PREGNANCY

BACKGROUND

- 2–3% of births (increasing due to artificial reproductive technology)
- 98% twins; overall risk of twins 1:89; 80% twins dizygous

DIAGNOSIS

History

- Suspect Dx if excessive sx of pregnancy
- *Risk factors* (dizygous): black race, family history, increased age & parity, artificial reproductive technology (*Note:* monozygous twinning random event in 1:300 pregnancies; increases 2- to 3-fold w/ in vitro fertilization)

Physical examination

- Suspect Dx if uterine size > dates

Diagnostic tests

- *Laboratory tests:* consider Dx if significantly increased human chorionic gonadotropin, maternal serum alpha-fetoprotein
- *Imaging tests:* ultrasound to confirm Dx, check chorionicity

DIFFERENTIAL DIAGNOSIS

- Incorrect dates
- Uterine fibroids
- Polyhydramnios
- Macrosomic fetus

COMPLICATIONS

- Antepartum complications develop in 80% multiples vs. 30% singletons
- *Maternal complications:* anemia, hyperemesis, preterm labor, preterm premature rupture of membranes, preeclampsia, gestational diabetes, previa, postpartum hemorrhage
- *Fetal complication:* preterm birth, fetal abnormalities, intrauterine growth restriction (5–15% twins, 30% triplets), intrauterine fetal demise, poly/oligo sequence (incl. twin-twin transfusion syndrome in 15% of monochorionic twins), cord entanglement (1/25,000 births; 70% of mono/mono pregnancies), malpresentation

PROGNOSIS

- Perinatal mortality increases w/ monochorionic vs. dichorionic twins & is esp. high w/ mono/mono twins (>50% due to cord entanglement)

MANAGEMENT

General measures

- Early Dx
- Determine chorionicity
- Serial ultrasound for fetal growth, discordance

Specific treatment

- In dichorionic twins, risk of aneuploidy independent for each fetus; consider amniocentesis for "advanced maternal age" in women >=32 y at delivery
- Regular fetal testing if evidence of growth discordance
- For higher-order multiples, discuss multifetal pregnancy reduction to twins at 11–13 wk (6–8% procedure-related loss rate <24 wk, similar to spontaneous loss rate; controversial in triplets)
- Twin-twin transfusion syndrome: perinatal mortality 20–80%; Rx options incl. expectant Mx, serial amnioreduction, laser obliteration of placental vascular communications
- Mode of delivery depends on fetal number, presentation, gestational age/estimated fetal weight
- Recent evidence suggests increased rate of long-term neurologic damage to second twins delivered via a breech vaginal delivery

Contraindications

- Vaginal delivery contraindicated in nonvertex presenting twin, higher-order multiples

SUBSEQUENT MANAGEMENT

- Depends on specific pathology

MYASTHENIA GRAVIS

BACKGROUND

- Autoimmune disease characterized by weakness, fatigability of voluntary muscle (smooth muscle, myometrium relatively unaffected)
- *Prevalence:* 50–125/million population; 25,000 people affected in U.S.

DIAGNOSIS

History

- Sx subtle (generalized weakness, fatigue)
- *Risk factors:* female (2:1; peak incidence in 3rd decade of life), HLA-B8 antigen

Physical examination

- Confirm generalized weakness

Diagnostic tests

- *Laboratory tests:* consider checking acetylcholine receptor antibodies (87% (+); correlate poorly w/ severity)
- *Specific diagnostic tests:* neostigmine bromide (0.5 mg IV, recheck strength in 30 min) preferred over edrophonium chloride [Tensilon] test (associated w/ premature labor, abortion)
- *Imaging tests:* not indicated

DIFFERENTIAL DIAGNOSIS

- Congenital myasthenic syndromes
- Drug-induced myasthenia
- Hyperthyroidism
- Eaton-Lambert syndrome
- Botulism
- Progressive ophthalmoplegia

COMPLICATIONS

- *Maternal complications:* abortion, myasthenic crisis (no increase in infertility, preeclampsia, preterm delivery)
- *Fetal complications:* neonatal myasthenia (transient syndrome in 12–15% infants due to transplacental passage of IgG; sx include lethargy, poor suck, feeble cry, generalized weakness; develops in 1–4 d, subsides 2–6 wk)

PROGNOSIS

- Effect of pregnancy on myasthenia unpredictable
- Overall, 1/3 experience remission, 1/3 relapse/exacerbate, 1/3 stable

MANAGEMENT

General measures

- Myasthenia not an indication for pregnancy termination
- Neurology consult
- Avoid infection, medications (phenytoin, gentamicin, anesthetics, magnesium, meperidine, morphine) that exacerbate sx

Specific treatment

Antepartum Mx

- Continue anticholinesterase Rx (neostigmine, pyridostigmine)
- Azathioprine, corticosteroids if unresponsive
- Plasmapheresis, thymectomy as last resort

Intrapartum Mx

- Continue anticholinesterase Rx
- Serial evaluation for evidence of muscle weakness, exhaustion
- Consider elective shortening of 2nd stage to decrease fatigue assoc. w/ expulsive efforts
- Avoid magnesium for seizure prophylaxis

Contraindications

■ Anticholinesterase Rx not contraindication to breastfeeding

Side effects & complications of treatment

■ Pediatricians should be aware that anticholinesterase Rx may protect infant from neonatal myasthenia leading to delayed Dx

SUBSEQUENT MANAGEMENT

■ Symptomatic relapse most likely in puerperium

OBSTETRIC ULTRASOUND

BACKGROUND

■ Uses high-frequency sound waves (3.5–5 MHz for transabdominal; 5–7.5 MHz for transvaginal); higher frequency assoc. w/ better resolution but less tissue penetration
■ Interpretation of images requires operator experience

DIAGNOSIS

■ Indications for obstetric ultrasound:

History

■ Pain
■ Decreased fetal movement
■ Bleeding, to exclude ectopic, previa (cannot exclude abruption, only see retroplacental blood clot >300 mL)

Physical examination

■ Uterine size > or < dates
■ Suspected uterine or adnexal mass
■ Abnormal cervical examination
■ Unable to document fetal heart rate
■ Confirm malpresentation

Diagnostic tests
- Abnormal maternal serum alpha-fetoprotein
- Adjunct to amniocentesis, chorionic villus sampling, external cephalic version, fetal therapy

DIFFERENTIAL DIAGNOSIS
- Alternative imaging techniques: (1) abdominal x-ray (for skeletal exam for limb dysplasia); (2) MRI (as adjunct for detailed assessment of fetal CNS anatomy, placenta, myometrial invasion)

COMPLICATIONS
- No confirmed adverse effects to mother or fetus, aside from false-positive & false-negative Dx

PROGNOSIS
- Routine ultrasound in low-risk pregnancies has not been shown to definitively improve perinatal outcome (but will improve gestational age estimation & thereby lower induction rates, improve performance of multiple marker screening, detection of structural anomalies, multiple pregnancies)

MANAGEMENT
Ultrasound useful for:
- Determination of gestational age (<10 wk: CRL; 10–14 wk: BPD; >14 wk: BPD, abdominal circumference, femur length)
- Identification & assessment of fetal anomalies
- Identification & assessment of multiple gestation
- Determination of fetal growth
- Determination of fetal well-being
- Characterization of placentation

Minimal criteria for adequate exam:
1. *1st trimester:*
    ➢ Localize gestational sac

- ➤ Document fetal cardiac activity
- ➤ Document fetal number
- ➤ Record CRL
- ➤ Assess uterus, adnexa
2. *2nd/3rd trimester:*
- ➤ Document fetal cardiac activity
- ➤ Document fetal number
- ➤ Assess amniotic fluid
- ➤ Localize placenta
- ➤ Assess gestational age
- ➤ Assess fetal growth
- ➤ Evaluate uterus, adnexa
- ➤ Document (at minimum) integrity of fetal spine, stomach, bladder, cerebral ventricles, kidneys, cord insertion

SUBSEQUENT MANAGEMENT
- ▦ Confirmatory imaging studies after delivery, if indicated

---

OLIGOHYDRAMNIOS

BACKGROUND
- ▦ Refers to abnormally small amount of amniotic fluid around fetus
- ▦ Net amniotic fluid volume (AFV) reflects balance between production & absorption; in 3rd trimester, fetal urine primary source of amniotic fluid (800–1,000 mL/d at term)
- ▦ AFV maximal at 32–34 wk (750–800 mL), decreases to 600 mL at 40 wk, continues to decrease thereafter
- ▦ Complicates 5–8% of pregnancies

DIAGNOSIS
History
- ▦ Usually asymptomatic

■ Leakage of clear vaginal fluid may suggest premature rupture of membrane

Physical examination
■ Usually unhelpful
■ Fundal height may be less than expected for gestational age

Diagnostic tests
■ Oligohydramnios is a *sonographic* Dx defined as (1) total AFV <300 mL, (2) absence of single 2-cm vertical pocket, or (3) amniotic fluid index (sum of maximum vertical pocket of amniotic fluid in each of 4 quadrants of uterus [AFI]) <5 cm at term or <5th percentile for gestational age
■ Look for cause, incl. premature rupture of membranes
■ Careful fetal anatomic survey (for renal anomalies [eg, Potter syndrome, bladder outlet obstruction, urethral obstruction, renal dysplasia, ureteral reflux], cardiac anomalies, neural tube defects)
■ Abnormal umbilical artery Doppler velocimetry may suggest uteroplacental insufficiency

DIFFERENTIAL DIAGNOSIS
■ Premature rupture of membranes (accounts for 50% of oligohydramnios)
■ Uteroplacental insufficiency (preeclampsia, postterm pregnancy, abruption)
■ Congenital anomalies (cardiac, renal)
■ Infection
■ Secondary to drug therapy (ACE inhibitors, nonsteroidal anti-inflammatory drugs)
■ Twin-to-twin transfusion syndrome

COMPLICATIONS
■ *Maternal complications:* generally few maternal complications; intraamniotic infection may occur in the setting of

premature rupture of membranes; increased cesarean rate due to malpresentation, nonreassuring fetal testing
- Fetal complications depend on etiology, severity, & gestational age
- *Fetal complications:* amniotic band syndrome, pulmonary hypoplasia (if severe oligohydramnios <22–24 wk), musculoskeletal deformities (eg, clubfoot) due to uterine compression, malpresentation, prematurity, intrauterine growth restriction, stillbirth

PROGNOSIS
- AFV a marker of fetal well-being; normal AFV suggests adequate uteroplacental perfusion
- Oligohydramnios assoc. w/ increased perinatal morbidity & mortality at any gestational age
- Fetal prognosis depends on cause & gestational age at delivery

MANAGEMENT
General measures
- Antepartum Mx options limited, unless a structural defect (eg, posterior urethral valve in male infant) identified & amenable to in utero shunting
- Timing of delivery depends on gestational age, etiology, severity of oligohydramnios, & fetal well-being

Specific treatment
- Confirm Dx
- Exclude premature rupture of membranes
- Regular fetal testing (2x or 1x wk nonstress test &/or ultrasound examination for AFV, biophysical profile, umbilical artery Doppler velocimetry; serial ultrasound for fetal growth)
- Consider confirmation of fetal lung maturity prior to delivery if oligohydramnios severe & prolonged; consider corticosteroids if indicated

■ In labor, infusion of crystalloid solution into amniotic cavity (amnioinfusion) may improve abnormal fetal heart rate patterns, decrease cesarean delivery rate, & minimize neonatal meconium aspiration

SUBSEQUENT MANAGEMENT
■ Recurrence rate depends on cause

OPERATIVE VAGINAL DELIVERY

BACKGROUND
■ Refers to any operative procedure designed to expedite vaginal delivery (episiotomy, forceps, vacuum)

DIAGNOSIS
History
■ Review possible need for operative vaginal delivery antepartum

Physical examination
■ Confirm cervical dilatation, vertex presentation, position, station
■ Assess clinical pelvimetry

Diagnostic tests
■ Not routinely indicated

DIFFERENTIAL DIAGNOSIS
■ Consider immediate cesarean
■ Distinguish assisted delivery from TRIAL OF assisted delivery (in which attempt made in OR while preparing for cesarean)

COMPLICATIONS
■ *Maternal complications:* perineal injury (esp. forceps), failure to effect delivery

■ *Fetal complications:* facial bruising, laceration; cephalhematoma (esp. vacuum); facial nerve palsy, skull fractures, cervical spine injuries, intracranial hemorrhage rare

PROGNOSIS
■ Dependent on operator experience, classification of procedure:
  ➤ Outlet (vertex on perineum, scalp visible w/out separating labia, sagittal suture in anteroposterior orientation, rotation <=45 degrees)
  ➤ Low (station >=+2 cm, vertex not on pelvic floor)
  ➤ Mid (station <+2 cm, but head engaged)
  ➤ High (not included)

MANAGEMENT
General measures
■ No proven benefit of one instrument over another
■ Choice of instrument depends on indication, clinician preference, & experience

Specific treatment
■ *Indications* identical for forceps & vacuum:
  1. Maternal exhaustion, inadequate expulsive efforts, need to avoid pushing
  2. Nonreassuring fetal testing
  3. Prolonged 2nd stage (nullipara 3 h w/ regional anesthesia, 2 h w/o; multipara 2 h w/ regional anesthesia, 1 h w/o)
2. Empty bladder, adequate analgesia
3. Episiotomy not required
4. *Forceps:* apply sustained downward traction along pelvic curvature in concert w/ uterine contractions, maternal expulsive efforts
5. *Vacuum:* place cup over "median flexing point," increase suction to 500–600 mmHg before traction, release between contractions; abandon after 4 traction efforts if cup detaches 2x, no descent, undelivered in 20–25 min

Contraindications
- *Absolute:* membranes intact, cervix not fully dilated, previa
- *Relative:* prematurity, macrosomia, fetal coagulopathy, malpresentation

SUBSEQUENT MANAGEMENT
- Follow-up maternal perineal injury, neonatal complications

PARAPLEGIA

BACKGROUND
- 11,000 spinal cord injuries in U.S. annually (due primarily to trauma); 15–30% in women of reproductive age

DIAGNOSIS

History
- Usually precedes pregnancy
- Ask about complications (decubitus ulcers, UTIs, pulmonary infections, autonomic dysreflexia)

Physical examination
- Check level, extent of cord injury
- Women w/ cord transection >T10 have painless labors but cannot perceive premature contractions; to detect preterm labor, consider regular ultrasound exams for cervical length until 30–32 weeks, then perform weekly cervical exams thereafter; ask pt to palpate abdomen 2x daily (or home uterine monitor) after 28 wk

Diagnostic tests
- *Laboratory tests:* routine testing
- *Specific diagnostic tests:* check baseline renal, pulmonary function tests in 2nd trimester, if indicated
- *Imaging tests:* not indicated

DIFFERENTIAL DIAGNOSIS
- Other neurologic Dx (multiple sclerosis, myasthenia gravis)
- Guillain-Barré syndrome
- Peripheral nerve injury
- Polio

COMPLICATIONS
- *Maternal complications:* anemia, UTIs, pressure sores; fertility unaffected
- *Fetal complications:* unaffected
- *Autonomic dysreflexia:* rare, life-threatening event in 85% of women with transection $>=$T5/6; due to loss of cortical control over spinal reflexes through viable segments of cord below transection triggered by stimulus (full bladder, pelvic exam, contractions, urinary catheter); presents as acute headache, hypertension, bradycardia, sweating, flushing, tingling, nasal congestion, cardiac dysrhythmias, respiratory distress

PROGNOSIS
- Depends on cause, level, & extent of spinal cord injury

MANAGEMENT

General measures
- Supportive care (prevent ulcers, contractures)
- Neurology consultation
- Antenatal anesthesia consultation

Specific treatment
- Suppressive antibiotics if recurrent UTIs, self-catheterize
- Pregnancy may compromise resp. status; ventilatory support occasionally needed at end of pregnancy
- Consider anesthesia consultation prior to delivery
- Adequate anesthesia for labor, delivery
- Prevent autonomic dysreflexia (minimize exams, manipulations, T10 epidural analgesia to block afferent stimuli); if occurs, control BP & sx, immediate cesarean

Contraindications

■ No contraindication to vaginal delivery; reserve cesarean for routine obstetric indications

Follow-up

■ Postpartum visit 1–2 wk, increased risk postpartum depression

SUBSEQUENT MANAGEMENT

■ Long-term neurology follow-up

PARVOVIRUS B19

BACKGROUND

■ Single-stranded DNA virus that causes fifth disease (erythema infectiosum)
■ Transmission by hand-to-mouth contact & respiratory secretions
■ Incubation period 5–10 d (infectious period usually past once clinical manifestations present)

DIAGNOSIS

History

■ History of exposure to fifth disease (40–50% of reproductive-age women have not previously been infected; in susceptible women, exposure results in seroconversion in 50–70% of cases if contact is household member & 20% if exposure occurs at school)
■ *Risk factors:* female gender, white race, age <30 y, contact w/ children 5–18 y old in home or workplace, teachers & daycare providers who have contact w/ younger children

Physical examination

■ Fifth disease is a common, self-limiting illness of childhood presenting w/ reticular facial & truncal rash, mild upper

respiratory tract sx, & low-grade fever; adults may develop self-limiting arthropathy
■ Characteristic clinical feature facial ("slapped-cheek") rash

Diagnostic tests
■ Maternal infection can be confirmed by serologic testing or direct visualization of viral particles in infected tissues
■ Fetal infection can be confirmed by detection of viral particles or DNA in fetal serum, amniotic fluid, placenta, or autopsy tissues; however, invasive prenatal testing not routinely recommended

DIFFERENTIAL DIAGNOSIS
■ Extensive differential Dx, incl. other viral infections

COMPLICATIONS
■ *Maternal complications:* transient aplastic crisis, cardiac failure (rare)
■ *Fetal complications:* anemia (due to parvovirus-induced bone marrow suppression), nonimmune hydrops (assoc. w/ fetal HCT <15%), stillbirth, spontaneous abortion
■ Parvovirus B19 is not a teratogen

PROGNOSIS
■ Transplacental passage of parvovirus B19 high (33%), but risk of fetal morbidity & mortality low (estimated 3% for household contact, <1% for school contact)
■ Serious fetal sequelae occur w/ infection <20 wk; if fetus survives, long-term development appears to be normal (but data limited)

MANAGEMENT
General measures
■ Rx primarily supportive
■ No effective Rx & no vaccine

Specific treatment
- Confirm maternal infection
- Identify source of exposure
- Serial antepartum fetal surveillance (weekly ultrasound x 10–14 wk) looking for development of nonimmune hydrops; after 14 wk, likelihood of parvovirus-mediated bone marrow suppression leading to anemia & nonimmune hydrops minimal
- Consider use of noninvasive ultrasound testing (middle cerebral artery peak velocity) to identify fetuses w/ anemia
- Should hydrops develop, Mx limited to either immediate delivery if gestational age favorable or percutaneous umbilical blood sampling to confirm Dx, exclude other causes, & (possibly) perform intrauterine blood transfusion to correct anemia & reverse hydropic changes

Prevention
- Avoid exposure if susceptible
- No vaccine or immune globulin available

SUBSEQUENT MANAGEMENT
- Antiparvovirus B19 IgM disappears w/in months; IgG persists for life
- Nonimmune fetal hydrops due to acute parvovirus B19 infection does not recur in subsequent pregnancies

---

PLACENTA ACCRETA

BACKGROUND
- Refers to abnormal attachment of placental villi to uterus
- *Classification:* abnormal attachment of placenta to myometrium (accreta), invasion into myometrium (increta), or penetration through myometrium (percreta)
- Placenta accreta is most common (1/2,500 deliveries)

DIAGNOSIS

History
- Usually unhelpful
- *Risk factors:* prior uterine surgery, placenta previa (risk of significant accreta w/ previa 5%; increases to 25% w/ previa & prior cesarean, >50% w/ 2 or more prior cesareans), smoking, grandmultiparity

Physical examination
- Clinical Dx w/ inability to remove placenta, excessive blood loss after delivery

Diagnostic tests
- *Laboratory tests:* check baseline CBC, PT/PTT once Dx made
- *Specific diagnostic tests tests:* identification of villi on cystoscopy confirms Dx of percreta
- *Imaging tests:* antenatal ultrasound, MRI may suggest Dx; little value in acute setting

DIFFERENTIAL DIAGNOSIS
- Retained placental fragments
- Other causes of postpartum hemorrhage (uterine atony, lower genital tract lacerations, uterine rupture, coagulopathy)

COMPLICATIONS
- *Maternal complications:* shock, blood transfusion, death, Asherman's syndrome, sterility
- *Fetal complications:* prematurity

PROGNOSIS
- Depends on early Dx, prompt & appropriate Mx

MANAGEMENT

General measures
- Monitor vital signs, O_2
- Anesthesia consult, IV access

- Correct anemia/coagulopathy
- Plan delivery w/ multidisciplinary team in tertiary care center, blood available

Specific treatment
- Consider preop. catheterization of hypogastric arteries
- Attempt conservative surgery (manual removal of placenta, D&C, ? uterine packing)
- May require further surgical Mx:
- Explorative laparotomy (consider vertical incision)
- Bilateral uterine artery ligation (O'Leary stitch)
- Bilateral hypogastric (internal iliac) artery ligation to decrease perfusion pressure by 50%
- Hysterectomy
- Bladder/bowel resection (percreta)
- If time permits, consider angiography & embolization
- Central hemodynamic monitoring, if needed
- Uterotonic & antibiotic Rx, as indicated
- Methotrexate Rx of retained placenta controversial

Side effects & complications of treatment
- Risks of blood component Rx include transfusion reaction, infection (hepatitis)

SUBSEQUENT MANAGEMENT
- Increase in abnormal placentation in future pregnancies

PLACENTA PREVIA

BACKGROUND
- Refers to implantation of placenta over internal cervical os in advance of fetal presenting part
- Classified according to degree to which placenta covers os (complete, partial, marginal)
- Complicates 1 in 200 pregnancies
- Accounts for 20% of all antepartum hemorrhage

DIAGNOSIS

History

- Painless, bright-red vaginal bleeding
- Confirm gestational age (Dx should ideally be made >28 wk once lower uterine segment has formed)
- *Risk factors:* multiparity, advanced maternal age, prior placenta previa, prior cesarean delivery, smoking

Physical examination

- Confirm bright-red vaginal bleeding (avoid pelvic exam in women w/ antepartum hemorrhage until placenta previa excluded)
- Evaluate hemodynamic status of mother
- Document fetal well-being (bleeding maternal & does not usually compromise fetal well-being)
- Confirm fetal presentation (malpresentation common, as placenta prevents engagement of presenting part)

Diagnostic tests

- *Laboratory tests:* check CBC, type & screen, coagulation studies (if indicated)
- *Imaging studies:* ultrasound can accurately diagnose placenta previa; may be incidental finding on midtrimester ultrasound

DIFFERENTIAL DIAGNOSIS

- Placental abruption (30% of antepartum hemorrhage)
- Vasa previa (rare)
- Other causes: early labor, genital tract lesion (cervical polyps, erosion) (50%)

COMPLICATIONS

- *Maternal:* placenta accreta occurs in 5–15% of pregnancies w/ placenta previa, 25% w/ previa & 1 prior cesarean, >50% w/ previa & 2 prior cesareans
- *Neonatal:* malpresentation, preterm birth; not assoc. w/ intrauterine growth restriction

PROGNOSIS

- Depends on extent of bleeding & gestational age

MANAGEMENT

General measures

- Maximize fetal maturation while minimizing risk to mother & fetus

Specific treatment

- Outpatient Mx may be possible for women w/ single small bleed who can maintain bedrest & proximity to hospital
- Elective cesarean recommended for complete previa at 36 wk after documentation of fetal lung maturity
- Vaginal delivery rarely appropriate but may be indicated in setting of intrauterine fetal demise, previable delivery, lethal fetal anomalies, or advanced labor w/ engagement of fetal head & minimal vaginal bleeding
- A "double set-up exam" in labor may be appropriate in rare circumstances when ultrasound cannot exclude placenta previa & patient strongly motivated for vaginal delivery (performed in OR w/ surgical anesthesia & 2 surgical teams; one team scrubbed & ready for immediate cesarean in event of hemorrhage or fetal distress; other team performs gentle bimanual exam initially of vaginal fornices & then cervical os)
- RhoGAM, if indicated

Contraindications

- Contraindications to expectant Mx: nonreassuring fetal testing, maternal hemodynamic instability, excessive vaginal bleeding
- Immediate cesarean may be required under these circumstances regardless of gestational age

Follow-up care

- Placenta previa may resolve w/ time, thus permitting vaginal delivery; follow-up ultrasound examination thus recommended (only 5% of previa identified by ultrasound in midtrimester persist to term)

■ Most episodes of bleeding not life-threatening, & delivery can be safely delayed in most cases

SUBSEQUENT MANAGEMENT

■ Placenta previa increases risk of previa in subsequent pregnancy

---

PLACENTAL ABRUPTION

BACKGROUND

■ Refers to premature separation of placenta from uterine wall
■ Complicates 1 in 120 pregnancies

DIAGNOSIS

History

■ Symptoms may include vaginal bleeding (80%), uterine contractions (35%), abdominal tenderness (70%), with or without nonreassuring fetal testing (50%)

■ *Risk factors:* hypertension (chronic hypertension, preeclampsia, eclampsia), prior placental abruption, trauma, smoking, cocaine, uterine anomaly, fibroids, multiparity, advanced maternal age, prolonged premature rupture of membranes (15% have underlying placental abruption), rapid decompression of an overdistended uterus (eg, as in multiple pregnancy, polyhydramnios), bleeding diathesis/thrombophilia

Physical examination

■ Confirm vaginal bleeding (*Note:* amount of bleeding may not be reliable indicator of severity of condition, since up to 20% of abruptions may be concealed without evidence of vaginal bleeding)

■ Uterine tenderness suggests extravasation of blood into myometrium (Couvelaire uterus)

- Serial measurements of fundal height may be useful to monitor large retroplacental blood collections
- Port-wine discoloration of amniotic fluid suggests the Dx

Diagnostic tests
- Placental abruption is a *clinical* Dx
- *Imaging tests:* ultrasound may reveal retroplacental clot (>=300 mL necessary for ultrasound visualization), retromembranous clot, or intraamniotic bleeding; will also exclude placenta previa; findings may be normal

DIFFERENTIAL DIAGNOSIS
- Placenta previa (20% of antepartum hemorrhage)
- Vasa previa (rare)
- Other: early labor, genital tract lesions (cervical polyps, erosion) (50%)

COMPLICATIONS
- *Maternal complications:* maternal mortality (due to hemorrhage, renal failure, cardiac failure) ranges from 0.5–5%. Significant coagulopathy seen in 10% of cases, esp. in setting of severe abruption w/ massive hemorrhage & fetal demise
- *Fetal complications:* intrauterine fetal death occurs in 10–35% of cases due primarily to fetal hypoxia, exsanguination, & complications of prematurity. Abruption also assoc. w/ increased rate of congenital anomalies & intrauterine growth restriction

PROGNOSIS
- Depends on underlying cause, extent of abruption, gestational age, & presence of complications (eg, coagulopathy)

MANAGEMENT
General measures
- Hospitalization indicated to evaluate maternal & fetal condition
- Confirm diagnosis by ultrasound if possible

- Exclude other causes of antepartum hemorrhage, esp. placenta previa

Specific treatment
- Mode & timing of delivery depend on condition & gestational age of fetus, condition of mother, & state of cervix
- In setting of maternal hemodynamic instability, aggressive blood & volume replacement should be initiated. Invasive hemodynamic monitoring & immediate cesarean may be necessary
- If the abruption is mild & pregnancy is remote from term, expectant management may be appropriate

Contraindications
- Placental abruption is a relative contraindication to tocolysis

SUBSEQUENT MANAGEMENT
- Placental abruption may recur in a subsequent pregnancy; risk depends on underlying cause, gestational age, & degree of abruption
- Recurrence rate is around 10% after 1 abruption, 25% after 2 abruptions
- Consider thrombophilia work-up

PNEUMONIA

BACKGROUND
- Incidence: 1–3/1,000 pregnancies
- Most common in 2nd/3rd trimesters
- Gravid uterus impinging on diaphragmatic excursion might impair clearing of secretions & predispose to pneumonia
- Causative organisms for "typical" pneumonia: *Streptococcus pneumoniae, Haemophilus influenzae*; for "atypical" pneumonia: *Mycoplasma pneumoniae*, viral, *Chlamydia pneumoniae*

DIAGNOSIS

History
- May be preceded by URTI
- Typical presentation incl. acute onset of chills, fever, productive cough
- May present w/ gradual onset of sx, headache, nonproductive cough

Physical examination
- Fever
- Crackles, dullness to percussion, egophony on respiratory exam
- O_2 saturation may be decreased

Diagnostic tests
- Dx requires high index of clinical suspicion
- Check CBC w/ differential
- Consider blood culture, purified protein derivative
- Sputum Gram stain & culture
- Chest x-ray (posteroanterior, lateral views) may show lobar alveolar consolidation ("typical") or interstitial infiltration ("atypical" pneumonia)

DIFFERENTIAL DIAGNOSIS
- Pulmonary embolism
- Appendicitis
- Bronchitis
- Asthma flare
- Tuberculosis
- HIV

COMPLICATIONS
- *Maternal complications:* sepsis, preterm labor & delivery
- *Fetal complications:* preterm birth

PROGNOSIS
- Prognosis good w/ prompt Dx & appropriate Rx

MANAGEMENT

General measures

■ Inpatient management (outpatient Rx not appropriate in pregnancy)

■ Aggressive hydration

■ Antipyretic, pain control as needed

■ Oxygen supplementation to keep O_2 saturation >95%

Specific treatment

■ Appropriate antibiotic Rx for community-acquired pneumonia incl. (1) ceftriaxone 1–2 g IV q24h plus erythromycin 500 mg po/IV q6h (or doxycycline 100 mg po/IV q12h); (2) azithromycin 500 mg IV q24h, then 250 mg po × 7 d; (3) amoxicillin/clavulanic acid 875/125 mg po bid × 14 d plus erythromycin 500 mg po/IV q6h (or doxycycline 100 mg po q12h)

■ Appropriate Rx for suspected aspiration pneumonia incl. (1) 3rd or 4th generation cephalosporin; (2) penicillin plus a beta-lactamase inhibitor

■ Suspected viral infection requires only supportive care

SUBSEQUENT MANAGEMENT

■ Routine respiratory precautions

■ Future pregnancies rarely affected

POLYHYDRAMNIOS

BACKGROUND

■ Abnormally large amount of amniotic fluid around fetus

■ Net amniotic fluid volume (AFV) reflects balance between production & absorption; in 3rd trimester, fetal urine primary source of amniotic fluid (800–1,000 mL/ d at term)

■ AFV is maximal at 32–34 wk (750–800 mL), decreases to 600 mL at 40 wk, continues to decrease thereafter

■ Occurs in 0.5–1.5% of pregnancies

DIAGNOSIS

History
- Usually asymptomatic
- May present w/ rapid increase in abdominal girth, weight gain, dyspnea, swelling of lower extremities & vulva

Physical examination
- Suspect Dx when fundal height significantly greater than expected for gestational age or difficulty feeling fetal parts

Diagnostic tests
- Polyhydramnios a *sonographic* Dx defined as (1) total AFV >2 L, (2) single vertical pocket >=10 cm, or (3) an amniotic fluid index (sum of maximum vertical pocket of amniotic fluid in each of 4 quadrants of the uterus [AFI]) >25 cm at term or >95th percentile for gestational age
- Blood tests for maternal disorders, including diabetes mellitus (AFV directly related to glycemic control), isoimmunization
- Ultrasound examination to identify cause, incl. twin pregnancy, fetal anatomic survey for cardiac anomalies, cystic adenomatoid lung deformity, placental abnormalities (chorioangioma), GI obstruction; defects in swallowing (eg, achalasia, CNS anomalies, tracheoesophageal fistula) may be suspected but often difficult to diagnose antepartum

DIFFERENTIAL DIAGNOSIS
- Polyhydramnios seen in 50–75% of cases of hydrops fetalis
- Twin-to-twin transfusion syndrome
- Placental anomaly (chorioangioma)
- Fetal aneuploidy (esp. if polyhydramnios occurs in setting of intrauterine growth restriction)

COMPLICATIONS
- *Maternal complications:* antepartum uterine overdistention may result in mechanical complications such as dyspnea,

refractory edema of lower extremities, vulva, & abdominal wall; preterm labor; preterm premature rupture of membranes; increased cesarean delivery rate due to malpresentation &/or dysfunctional labor; postpartum hemorrhage

■ *Fetal complications:* unstable lie leading to malpresentation in labor, preterm premature rupture of membranes w/ cord prolapse, prematurity, stillbirth

PROGNOSIS

■ AFV a marker of fetal well-being; normal AFV suggests adequate uteroplacental perfusion

■ Polyhydramnios assoc. w/ increased perinatal morbidity & mortality at any gestational age; also assoc. w/ increased maternal morbidity

■ Fetal prognosis depends on cause & gestational age at delivery

MANAGEMENT

General measures

■ Antepartum Mx options limited

■ Nonsteroidal antiinflammatory drugs (indomethacin) can decrease fetal urine output & thereby AFV but may cause premature closure of fetal ductal arteriosus

■ Removal of fluid by amniocentesis may be indicated to relieve maternal discomfort but is only transiently effective (fluid reaccumulates w/in 48–72 h), may be assoc. w/ placental abruption (esp. if >2 L of fluid removed), & amniocentesis can cause premature rupture of membranes

■ Timing of delivery depends on gestational age, etiology, severity of polyhydramnios, & fetal well-being

Specific treatment

■ Confirm Dx

■ Attempt to identify cause (50–60% of cases have no known cause)

- Regular fetal testing (incl. serial ultrasound examination for fetal growth)
- In labor, controlled amniotomy may decrease complications resulting from rapid decompression of uterus (cord prolapse, placental abruption)

SUBSEQUENT MANAGEMENT
- Recurrence rate depends on cause

POSTPARTUM DEPRESSION

BACKGROUND
- Characterized by feelings of hopelessness & sadness w/ or w/o vegetative sx (insomnia, loss of appetite, weight loss)
- Peak onset of sx 2–3 mo postpartum, usually resolves spontaneously w/in 6–12 mo
- Incidence: 8–15% of all postpartum women

DIAGNOSIS
History
- Ask about prior postpartum depression, known psychiatric Dx (depression, bipolar disease), current meds
- *Risk factors:* history of depression (30% risk of postpartum depression), prior postpartum depression (70–85% risk)

Physical examination
- Usually unhelpful

Diagnostic tests
- *Laboratory tests:* none indicated
- *Specific diagnostic tests:* consider tests to exclude other Dx (eg, thyroid-stimulating hormone, EEG, lumbar puncture)
- *Imaging tests:* consider head CT or MRI to exclude mass lesion (esp. if localizing sx or focal neurologic signs present)

■ *Screening tests:* ask all pts at 6-wk postpartum visit about postpartum depression

DIFFERENTIAL DIAGNOSIS
■ Mild transient depression, also known as "postpartum blues" (very common immediately after delivery, occurring in >50% of women)
■ Exacerbation of major depression, bipolar disorder
■ Postpartum psychosis
■ Hypothyroidism
■ Temporal lobe epilepsy

COMPLICATIONS
■ *Maternal complications:* severe depression, self-inflicted injury, suicide, complications of Rx
■ *Fetal complications:* neonate may be at risk of neglect, abuse

PROGNOSIS
■ Usually short-lived & self-limiting

MANAGEMENT
General measures
■ In women w/ known psychiatric Dx, meds should be continued in pregnancy; in general, risk of relapse poses much greater threat to pregnancy than continued Rx

Specific treatment
■ Supportive care, regular follow-up usually all that is necessary
■ If drug Rx necessary, follow basic guidelines: (1) single agent, (2) lowest effective dose, (2) avoid excessive sedating agents to minimize neonatal sedation
■ Electroconvulsant therapy (ECT) rarely indicated

Follow-up care
■ Consider long-term psychology/psychiatry follow-up

SUBSEQUENT MANAGEMENT

- Future pregnancies increase risk of postpartum depression

POSTPARTUM HEMORRHAGE

BACKGROUND

- Traditionally defined as estimated blood loss $>=500$ mL; more recently as bleeding resulting in 10% decreased HCT or blood transfusion
- Incidence: 10–15% (4% w/ vaginal, 6–8% w/ cesarean)
- Classified as early (<24 h), late (>24 h but <6 wk postpartum)

DIAGNOSIS

History

- Ask about prior postpartum hemorrhage, excessive blood loss at surgery, menorrhagia
- Drugs (anticoagulants, aspirin)
- Family Hx of bleeding diathesis

Physical examination

- *Clinical* Dx w/ excessive blood loss after delivery

Diagnostic tests

- *Laboratory tests:* check CBC, PT/PTT
- *Specific diagnostic tests:* none
- *Imaging tests:* little value in acute setting

DIFFERENTIAL DIAGNOSIS

Causes:

- *Uterine atony:* increases risk w/ uterine overdistension, grand-multiparity, relaxants (magnesium, anesthetics, nitroglycerin)
- Retained placental fragments
- *Genital tract lacerations:* increases w/ macrosomia, episiotomy, forceps delivery, precipitous delivery

- *Uterine rupture:* 1/2,000 births; increases w/ prior uterine surgery, oxytocin
- *Uterine inversion:* 1/2,500 births; increases w/ excessive cord traction, manual removal of placenta, abnormal placentation
- *Abnormal placentation:* 1/2,500 births; increases w/ prior uterine surgery, previa, smoking
- *Coagulopathy,* congenital (vWd; 2/10,000 pregnancies), acquired (DIC, sepsis, anticoagulants, amniotic fluid embolism, immune thrombocytopenic purpura)
- *Infection* (endometritis)

COMPLICATIONS
- *Maternal complications:* blood transfusion, shock, hysterectomy, death
- *Fetal complications:* none

PROGNOSIS
- Depends on cause, Mx

MANAGEMENT
General measures
- Check hemodynamic status
- Anesthesia consult, large-bore IV access at multiple sites
- Stop bleeding, replace blood products

Specific treatment
- Rx uterine atony: IV/IM oxytocin 10–40 U; Cytotec (misoprostol) 1,000 mg PR × 1; methylergonovine 0.2 mg IM q2–4h × 3; 15-methyl PGF2-alpha (Hemabate) 25 mcg IM q15–90 min × 8; PGE2 (dinoprostone) 20 mg PR q2h × 3; unsuccessful, laparotomy w/ hypogastric, uterine artery ligation
- D&C for retained products
- Repair of genital tract laceration, uterine rupture; hysterectomy, if necessary
- Antibiotics, as indicated

SUBSEQUENT MANAGEMENT
- Future pregnancies increase risk of postpartum hemorrhage
- Consider thrombophilia work-up

POSTPARTUM PSYCHOSIS

BACKGROUND
- Characterized by development of psychotic sx after delivery; peak onset 10–14 d postpartum
- Incidence: 1–2/1,000 live births

DIAGNOSIS

History
- Ask about prior postpartum depression or psychosis, known psychiatric Dx (depression, bipolar disease), current medications
- *Risk factors:* younger age, primiparity, personal or family history of mental illness, prior postpartum psychosis (25–30% risk)

Physical examination
- Usually unhelpful

Diagnostic tests
- *Laboratory tests:* none indicated
- *Specific diagnostic tests:* consider tests to exclude other Dx (eg, thyroid-stimulating hormone, EEG, rapid plasma reagin (RPR), lumbar puncture)
- *Imaging tests:* consider head CT or MRI to exclude mass lesion (esp. if localizing sx or focal neurologic signs present)

DIFFERENTIAL DIAGNOSIS
- Mild transient depression, also known as "postpartum blues" (very common immediately after delivery, occurring in >50% of women)

- Postpartum depression
- Exacerbation of major depression, bipolar disorder
- Hypothyroidism
- Temporal lobe epilepsy
- Cryptococcal meningitis
- Tertiary syphilis

COMPLICATIONS
- *Maternal complications:* severe depression, self-inflicted injury, suicide, complications of Rx
- *Fetal complications:* neonate may be at risk of neglect, abuse

PROGNOSIS
- Usually short-lived & self-limiting

MANAGEMENT

General measures
- In women w/ known psychiatric Dx, continue meds in pregnancy; in general, risk of relapse poses greater threat to pregnancy than continued Rx

Specific treatment
- Hospitalization, pharmacologic Rx, &/or electroconvulsant therapy may be necessary
- Consider psychiatric consultation
- If drug Rx necessary, follow basic guidelines: (1) single agent, (2) lowest effective dose, (2) avoid excessive sedating agents to minimize neonatal sedation
- In general, mood-stabilizing drugs compatible w/ breastfeeding

Follow-up care
- Regular (weekly) follow-up
- Consider long-term psychiatric follow-up

SUBSEQUENT MANAGEMENT
- Recurrence of postpartum psychosis in subsequent pregnancy high (25–30%)

POSTTERM (PROLONGED) PREGNANCY

BACKGROUND
- Refers to pregnancy >=42.0 wk (294 d) from last menstrual period
- Complicates 10% of singleton pregnancies; 4% continue >=43 wk in absence of obstetric intervention

DIAGNOSIS

History
- Accurate dating critical to Dx
- *Risk factors:* primiparity, prior postterm pregnancy, family history of prolonged pregnancy; less common assoc. incl. anencephaly (w/o polyhydramnios), placental sulfatase deficiency, male fetus
- Most postterm pregnancies have no known cause

Physical examination
- Routine exam, incl. estimated fetal weight & clinical pelvimetry

Diagnostic tests
- Consider early ultrasound for dating
- Assessment of fetal well-being

DIFFERENTIAL DIAGNOSIS
- Incorrect dating
- Term "postdates" poorly defined & best avoided

COMPLICATIONS

- *Maternal complications:* increase in cesarean delivery (secondary to labor dystocia), 3rd/4th degree perineal lacerations, postpartum hemorrhage, endometritis
- *Fetal complications:* increased stillbirth & neonatal mortality, fetal dysmaturity syndrome (intrauterine growth restriction secondary to postterm uteroplacental insufficiency), meconium aspiration, complications of macrosomia (shoulder dystocia, brachial plexus injury), short-term neonatal complications (respiratory insufficiency, hypoglycemia, seizures)

PROGNOSIS

- Increases maternal & perinatal mortality & morbidity
- No differences in IQ or physical milestones at 1 y of age

MANAGEMENT

General measures

- Delivery generally recommended when risks to fetus greater than those faced by neonate after birth; in high-risk women, the balance shifts in favor of delivery at 38–39 wk
- Mx of low-risk pregnancies more controversial & depends on results of antepartum fetal assessment, cervical exam, gestational age, & maternal preference. However, balance may begin to shift by 41 weeks. Among twin gestations, the balance of risk may shift after 38 weeks.

Specific treatment

- Consider antepartum fetal testing (nonstress test, biophysical profile, amniotic fluid volume, contraction stress test) starting at 41 wk; usually performed 1x or 2x/wk; no single test has been shown superior
- Delivery recommended if evidence of oligohydramnios or fetal compromise
- Induction of labor at term in multipara & nullipara w/ favorable cervix does not increase risk of cesarean delivery

- In nullipara w/ unfavorable cervix at 41 wk, expectant Mx & induction of labor both acceptable Mx alternatives; however, routine induction of labor w/ newer cervical ripening agents shown to result in fewer failed & serial inductions, lower fetal & maternal morbidity, shorter hospital stay, & lower medical cost than expectant Mx
- Postterm fetus at high risk of intrapartum complications (fetal heart rate abnormalities, passage of meconium); continuous fetal heart rate monitoring therefore required in labor

Prevention
- Risks of routine induction of labor (specifically cesarean delivery) at 41 wk in era of cervical ripening agents lower than previously reported; although low, risk of fetal death at 41+ wk not zero, even w/ carefully monitored postterm pregnancies
- Routine induction of labor at 41 wk prevents fetal & maternal complications assoc. w/ postterm pregnancy

SUBSEQUENT MANAGEMENT
- Prolonged pregnancy may recur; as such, accurate determination of gestational age should be made early in subsequent pregnancies

---

PREECLAMPSIA

BACKGROUND
- Multisystem disorder specific to human pregnancy; disease of placenta
- Complicates 6–8% of pregnancies
- Preeclampsia *clinical* Dx made after 20 wk w/ 3 elements: new-onset hypertension (BP >=140/90 mmHg), proteinuria (>300 mg/24 h or >=1+ on clean-catch urine in absence of UTI), ± nondependent edema
- Classified as "mild" or "severe" (no "moderate" category)

DIAGNOSIS

History
- Usually asymptomatic
- May present w/ increasing edema, weight gain, sx of severe preeclampsia (headache, visual changes, RUQ pain)
- *Risk factors:* nulliparity, extremes of maternal age, African-American race, coexisting maternal disease (chronic hypertension, renal disease, diabetes)

Physical examination
- Check BP, proteinuria, urine output
- Evaluate maternal neurologic & hemodynamic status

Diagnostic tests
- No reliable diagnostic or screening test (roll-over test, uterine artery notching in early pregnancy may predict women at risk)
- Check liver & renal function tests, platelet count, proteinuria

DIFFERENTIAL DIAGNOSIS
- Other hypertensive disorders of pregnancy (chronic hypertension, pregnancy-induced hypertension)
- Other maternal diseases (SLE flare, primary renal disease, pheochromocytoma)
- Complication of drug therapy (eg, long-term corticosteroid therapy)
- Drug withdrawal, esp. cocaine
- False-positive BP measurement (BP cuff too small, pt not at rest)

COMPLICATIONS
- *Maternal complications:* HELLP (hemolysis, elevated liver enzymes, low platelets) syndrome, thrombocytopenia, coma or seizures (eclampsia), renal failure, cardiac failure, pulmonary edema, placental abruption, DIC, stroke, maternal mortality
- *Fetal complications:* uteroplacental insufficiency & intrauterine growth restriction, stillbirth, prematurity

PROGNOSIS

■ Preeclampsia & its complications almost always resolve following delivery (except stroke); postpartum diuresis >4 L/d most accurate clinical indicator of resolution

■ Fetal prognosis dependent largely on gestational age at delivery

MANAGEMENT

General measures

■ Delivery *only* effective Rx

■ BP control important to prevent stroke but does not affect course of preeclampsia

■ Timing & route of delivery depend on severity of preeclampsia, condition & gestational age of fetus, condition of mother

Specific treatment

■ Confirm Dx

■ Mild preeclampsia should be managed expectantly as inpatient

■ Regular fetal testing (serial ultrasound examinations for fetal growth, weekly-daily nonstress test after 32 wk)

■ Delivery generally recommended (1) in mild preeclampsia once favorable gestational age reached; (2) in severe preeclampsia regardless of gestational age (w/ exception of severe preeclampsia due to proteinuria or intrauterine growth restriction remote from term w/ good fetal testing; recent trend toward expectant Mx of severe preeclampsia by BP criteria alone <32 wk)

■ No proven benefit to cesarean delivery, but probability of vaginal delivery in pt w/ severe preeclampsia remote from term w/ unfavorable cervix only 14–20%

■ Magnesium sulfate (4–6 g IV load, 1–2 g/h infusion) should be given intrapartum & for >=24 h postpartum as seizure prophylaxis

Prevention

■ Despite promising early studies, low-dose acetylsalicylic & supplemental calcium do not prevent preeclampsia in high- or low-risk women

SUBSEQUENT MANAGEMENT

■ May be assoc. w/ chronic hypertension, cardiovascular disease, renal disease in later life
■ Recurrence rate ranges from 10–70%; depends on gestational age at presentation & severity of preeclampsia, with earlier presentations more likely to recur than term presentations

---

PREGESTATIONAL DIABETES

BACKGROUND

■ Due to insulin deficiency (type I, insulin-dependent) or increased peripheral insulin resistance (type II, noninsulin-dependent)
■ White classification developed in attempt to correlate severity of diabetes w/ pregnancy outcome
■ <1% of women of childbearing age

DIAGNOSIS

History

■ Confirm diabetes prior to pregnancy
■ Usually asymptomatic

Physical examination

■ Depends on severity of diabetes (ranges from no physical signs to hypertension, retinal vasculopathy)

Diagnostic tests

■ Serial blood glucose monitoring
■ Check HbA1c (glycosylated Hb, reflects glycemic control over prior 3 mo) prior to conception & in 1st trimester

DIFFERENTIAL DIAGNOSIS
- Gestational diabetes
- Isolated glycosuria w/o diabetes

COMPLICATIONS
- Pregestational diabetes is assoc. w/ significant maternal & perinatal mortality & morbidity
- *Maternal complications:* chronic hypertension, diabetic ketoacidosis, preeclampsia, spontaneous abortion, polyhydramnios, preterm labor, increased cesarean delivery, infection (pyelonephritis, postpartum endometritis)
- *Fetal complications:* congenital anomalies (correlates directly w/ periconceptional glycemic control), fetal macrosomia w/ or w/o birth injury, intrauterine growth restriction, stillbirth (50–90% mortality w/ diabetic ketoacidosis), unexplained late intrauterine fetal demise, neonatal hypoglycemia, delayed organ maturation (respiratory distress syndrome, neonatal hyperbilirubinemia)

PROGNOSIS
- Poor prognostic features: diabetic ketoacidosis, hypertension, pyelonephritis, vasculopathy, poor compliance
- Overall prognosis good w/ tight glycemic control

MANAGEMENT
General measures
- Women should be seen prior to conception; pregnancy complications such as congenital anomalies & spontaneous abortion correlate directly w/ degree of diabetic control at conception
- Tight glycemic control can decrease perinatal mortality from 20% to 3–5%
- In pregnancy, goal is to prevent maternal & fetal complications by maintaining blood glucose at desirable levels (fasting,

<95 mg/dL; 1 h postprandial, <140 mg/dL; 2 h postprandial, <120 mg/dL)

■ Diabetic diet (15 kcal/lb or 36 kcal/kg ideal body weight + 100 kcal per trimester given as 20% protein, 40–50% carbohydrate, 30–40% fat) recommended for all women

■ Oral hypoglycemic agents still being evaluated for safety and efficacy in pregnancy

■ Insulin Rx of choice (0.7–1.0 U/kg/d given as 2/3 in AM [60% NPH, 40% regular], 1/3 in PM [50% NPH/50% regular])

Specific treatment

■ Home monitoring of blood glucose qid; wkly follow-up; adjustment of insulin therapy as indicated

■ Ophthalmologic exam q trimester

■ Check thyroid-stimulating hormone (6% of women have concurrent thyroid dysfunction)

■ Detailed sonographic fetal anatomic survey at 18–22 wk

■ Weekly fetal testing after 32 wk; ultrasound for growth at 36–37 wk

■ Delivery should be achieved by 39–40 wk

■ Elective cesarean may be indicated if estimated fetal weight excessive (possibly >=4,500 g) because of risk of birth injury

■ Intrapartum Mx should include NPO, IV glucose (5% dextrose at 75–100 mL/h), q 1–2 h blood glucose estimations, & regular insulin IV or SC to maintain blood glucose levels at 100–120 mg/dL

■ Check neonatal blood glucose level w/in 1 h of birth

SUBSEQUENT MANAGEMENT

■ During first 48 h postpartum, women may have "honeymoon period" w/ decreased insulin requirement; glucose levels of 150–200 mg/dL can be tolerated during this period

■ Once pt able to eat, she can be back on her prepregnancy insulin regimen

PREGNANCY-INDUCED HYPERTENSION

BACKGROUND

- Effects of pregnancy on maternal cardiovascular system: blood volume increases 0.800 L by 12 wk (1.5 L in twins); BP decreases in early pregnancy (due primarily to decreased peripheral vascular resistance), hits nadir in midpregnancy, & returns to baseline by term
- Pregnancy-induced hypertension (PIH) refers to sustained elevation of BP>=140/90 in 3rd trimester (after 20 weeks) w/o evidence of preeclampsia in previously normotensive woman
- PIH (also known as transient, nonproteinuric, gestational hypertension) probably represents exaggerated physiologic response of maternal cardiovascular system to pregnancy. Physiology is likely distinctly different than that of preeclampsia.

DIAGNOSIS

History

- Usually asymptomatic
- May present w/ increased edema, headache
- *Risk factors:* prior PIH, advanced maternal age, family history

Physical examination

- Check BP (use appropriate-size BP cuff, pt should be sitting at rest, use disappearance of sounds [5th Korotkoff sound] for diastolic measurement in pregnancy)
- No signs of chronic hypertension (eg, retinal changes)

Diagnostic tests

- Remains *clinical* Dx based on serial BP measurements
- PIH is Dx of exclusion (after delivery, BP returns to normal w/o evidence of preeclampsia)

DIFFERENTIAL DIAGNOSIS

- Other hypertensive disorders of pregnancy (chronic hypertension, preeclampsia)
- Pheochromocytoma
- Complication of drug therapy (eg, long-term corticosteroid therapy)
- Drug withdrawal, esp. cocaine
- False-positive BP measurement (BP cuff too small, patient not at rest)

COMPLICATIONS

- Rarely assoc. w/ adverse maternal or fetal outcome (unless Dx preeclampsia)
- BP >=160/110 (may be assoc. w/ increased risk of maternal CVA) suggests Dx preeclampsia, not PIH

PROGNOSIS

- PIH does not progress to preeclampsia; however, BP elevation in 3rd trimester may be first sign of preeclampsia, & it may not be possible to distinguish clinically between PIH & preeclampsia until disease progresses further
- PIH resolves rapidly after delivery

MANAGEMENT

General measures

- Assess fetal & maternal well-being
- EXCLUDE PREECLAMPSIA (check liver function tests, platelet count, renal function, urinary output, 24-h urinary protein analysis)

Specific treatment

- Mode & timing of delivery depend on severity of hypertension, condition & gestational age of fetus, & condition of mother
- No antihypertensive therapy indicated unless elevation in BP severe enough to place pt at risk of CVA (usually regarded as >=160/110 mmHg), which is an indication for delivery

- PIH at term a relative indication for induction of labor, since up to 15% of such women ultimately shown to have preeclampsia
- Women w/ PIH & no evidence of preeclampsia do not require magnesium sulfate seizure prophylaxis in labor

SUBSEQUENT MANAGEMENT
- PIH tends to recur in subsequent pregnancies
- PIH is assoc. w/ increased risk of chronic hypertension in later life

PRENATAL DIAGNOSIS

BACKGROUND
- Designed to detect fetal structural, chromosomal, genetic, metabolic disorders prior to delivery
- *Incidence:* 2–3% births have major congenital anomalies, 5% have minor malformations
- 60–70% structural anomalies have no known cause

DIAGNOSIS

History
- Complete pt, family history, ethnic background
- *Risk factors:* advanced maternal age ($>=35$ y at delivery; 5–8% of births but 20–30% Down syndrome), prior affected pregnancy, drug/toxin exposure

Diagnostic tests
- *Routine testing:*
  - ➣ Nuchal translucency at 10–14 wk >95 percentile for crown-rump length
  - ➣ Maternal serum alpha-fetoprotein (MS-AFP) >2.5 MoM (multiples of the median) at 15–20 wk: neural tube defect (check ultrasound; amniotic fluid alpha-fetoprotein, acetylcholinesterase activity)

➤ Serum "quad screen" (MS-AFP, human chorionic gonado-tropin, estriol, inhibin-A) at 15–20 wk adjusts age-related risk for aneuploidy
➤ Sonographic structural survey 18–22 wk
■ *Invasive testing:*
➤ Amniocentesis >15 wk for DNA analysis, karyotype, metabolic tests
➤ Chorionic villus sampling 10–12 wk for cytogenetic tests, DNA analysis, enzyme assays
➤ Percutaneous umbilical blood sampling >18 wk for kary-otype, check hematologic, immunologic, acid/base para-meters

DIFFERENTIAL DIAGNOSIS
■ *Chromosomal anomalies:*
➤ Autosomal: trisomy 21 (Down syndrome, 1/800 births); trisomy 18 (Edward); trisomy 13 (Patau)
➤ Sex chromosome: 45,X (Turner), 47,XXY (Klinefelter)
■ *Genetic disorders:*
➤ Autosomal dominant (70%): Huntington, neurofibroma-tosis, Marfan syndrome, achondroplasia
➤ Autosomal recessive (20%): Tay-Sachs, sickle cell, cystic fibrosis, beta-thalassemia, phenylketonuria
➤ X-linked recessive (5%): hemophilia, Duchenne
➤ X-linked dominant (rare): vitamin D-resistant rickets
➤ Multifactorial: neural tube defect, club feet, hydrocephaly, cleft lip/palate

COMPLICATIONS
■ *Maternal complications:* abruption, isoimmunization
■ *Fetal complications:* prematurity, stillbirth

PROGNOSIS
■ Depends on Dx

MANAGEMENT

General measures

- Mx options: pregnancy termination, further testing/Rx, delivery at tertiary care center
- Genetic counseling
- Pediatric surgery consultation
- RhoGAM, if indicated, to prevent isoimmunization

Side effects & complications of treatment

- Procedure-related loss rate: 1/270 for amniocentesis (increases <15 wk); 1–2% for chorionic villus sampling; 1–2% for percutaneous umbilical cord sampling (higher in fetuses with hydrops, intrauterine growth restriction)
- Chorionic villus sampling <=9 wk assoc. w/ limb reduction defects

SUBSEQUENT MANAGEMENT

- Recurrence rate depends on Dx

PRETERM LABOR

BACKGROUND

- Refers to labor <37 wk gestation
- Complicates 7–12% of deliveries; accounts for 85% of perinatal morbidity & mortality (excluding congenital abnormalities)
- 20% preterm births iatrogenic for maternal/fetal indications; 30% due to preterm premature rupture of membranes; 20% spontaneous preterm labor; 30% infection

DIAGNOSIS

History

- Symptoms of uterine contractions
  - ➤ Increased vaginal discharge
  - ➤ Spotting

> Sensation of pelvic pressure
- *Risk factors:* prior preterm birth, infection, African-American race, low socioeconomic status, advanced maternal age, multiple pregnancy, bleeding, smoking, uterine anomaly, smoking, cocaine; 50% of women delivering preterm have no risk factors

Physical examination
- Palpable uterine contractions; fever, maternal/fetal tachycardia, uterine tenderness may suggest intrauterine infection
- Progressive cervical effacement or/ & dilatation is prerequisite for Dx (or initial exam >=2 cm &/or >=80%)

Diagnostic tests
- Preterm labor *clinical* Dx
- Consider amniocentesis to exclude infection; wet smear to exclude preterm premature rupture of membranes, vaginal infection

DIFFERENTIAL DIAGNOSIS
- Preterm contractions
- Cervical insufficiency

COMPLICATIONS
- *Maternal complications:* increased cesarean delivery, infection
- *Fetal complications:* depend on gestational age at delivery & incl. neonatal death, respiratory distress syndrome, intraventricular hemorrhage, necrotizing enterocolitis, sepsis, hypoglycemia, jaundice, hypocalcemia

PROGNOSIS
- Perinatal outcome depends on cause, gestational age at delivery, & complications of prematurity

MANAGEMENT

General measures

- Confirm Dx (document both uterine contractions & cervical change)
- Look for cause: 30% of preterm labor due to intraamniotic infection; >50% no known cause
- Cesarean delivery for usual obstetric indications

Specific treatment

- Exclude contraindications to expectant Mx, tocolysis (intrauterine infection, nonreassuring fetal testing, bleeding, intrauterine fetal demise, lethal congenital anomaly; preterm premature rupture of membranes, bleeding relative contraindications)
- Bedrest, hydration commonly recommended but w/o proven efficacy
- Antenatal corticosteroids when indicated
- Short-term pharmacologic Rx cornerstone of Mx; no reliable data to show any agent can delay delivery for $>=48$ h
- No tocolytic agent clearly superior: (1) $MgSO_4$ 4–6 g IV bolus, 1–3 g/h IV infusion; (2) beta-adrenergic agonists (terbutaline 2 mcg/min IV or 0.25 mg SC q20 min; ritodrine 50 mcg/min IV or 5–10 mg IM q2–4h); (3) indomethacin 25–50 mg po q4–6h or 100 mg pr q12h; (4) newer agents (potassium channel openers, oxytocin receptor antagonists [atosiban], selective COX-2 inhibitors [meloxicam])
- Concurrent use of 2 or more agents not more effective, has increased side effects, & not recommended; sequential use of agents, however, may be effective
- Consider transfer to tertiary care center, if indicated

Prevention

- Several techniques have been used to predict preterm labor (risk factor analysis, home uterine monitoring, serial digital cervical exam) but have not been shown to decrease preterm birth, improve perinatal mortality

- Tests identifying women at increased risk of preterm birth: (1) cervical shortening on ultrasound, (2) biochemical tests (fetal fibronectin [99% of women w/ (–) test at 22–24 wk will be pregnant in 7 d, (+) test gives only 23% risk of delivery <35 wk]), (3) endocrine tests (salivary estriol >=2.1 ng/mL), (4) evidence of vaginal infection (esp. bacterial vaginosis)
- Maintenance tocolysis beyond 48 h (oral or IV) has no proven benefit but has significant risk & is not generally recommended

SUBSEQUENT MANAGEMENT
- Prior preterm birth a risk factor for preterm birth in subsequent pregnancy

---

PRETERM PROM

BACKGROUND
- Refers to rupture of membranes <37 wk prior to onset of labor
- Occurs in 33% of preterm deliveries
- If managed expectantly, 50% go into labor <24 h, 90% <1 wk

DIAGNOSIS
History
- Gush or persistent leakage of fluid from vagina
- May be increased uterine activity

Physical examination
- Confirm by speculum exam: vaginal pooling, leakage from cervix w/ Valsalva
- Limit bimanual exams (assoc. w/ increased infection)

Diagnostic tests
- *Laboratory tests:* vaginal pH >7.1 suggests rupture

- *Specific diagnostic tests:* ferning of vaginal fluid on glass slide suggests rupture; consider amnio-dye test if Dx equivocal (intraamniotic injection of dye, check tampon for leakage in 20–30 min)
- *Imaging tests:* oligohydramnios on ultrasound suggests Dx (normal fluid does not exclude Dx)

DIFFERENTIAL DIAGNOSIS
- Leakage of urine
- Vaginal infection
- Cervicitis
  - Cervical insufficiency

COMPLICATIONS
- *Maternal complications:* increased cesarean (due to cord prolapse, nonreassuring fetal testing), abruption (5–6%), chorioamnionitis (30–60%), postpartum endometritis (15%)
- *Fetal complications:* prematurity, malpresentation, stillbirth (1%), cord prolapse, neonatal sepsis (5%; 15–20% assoc. w/ clinical chorioamnionitis)

PROGNOSIS
- Related to cause of preterm PROM, gestational age

MANAGEMENT

General measures
- Check fetal presentation
- Exclude chorioamnionitis (temp >100.4 degrees F, fundal tenderness, maternal &/or fetal tachycardia); WBC generally unhelpful

Specific Rx
- Limit digital vaginal exams
- Antenatal corticosteroids if <32 wk; unclear benefit 32–34 wk
- Broad-spectrum antibiotic Rx (eg, IV ampicillin/erythromycin x 48 h, followed by po x 5 d) assoc. w/ increased latency, improved maternal/perinatal outcome

- Tocolytic Rx relatively contraindicated (unclear benefit, may delay delivery of compromised fetus)
- Intrapartum (not antepartum) group B *streptococcus* chemoprophylaxis, if indicated
- Routine fetal testing

Contraindications
- Contraindications to expectant Mx: chorioamnionitis, unstoppable preterm labor, nonreassuring fetal testing

Follow-up care
- If chorioamnionitis, Rx IV broad-spectrum antibiotics (incl. clindamycin) until 24–48 h afebrile

SUBSEQUENT MANAGEMENT
- Increased preterm PROM in future pregnancies (5–25%)
- Evaluate for cervical incompetence, if indicated

PUERPERAL HYSTERECTOMY

BACKGROUND
- Puerperal hysterectomy refers to removal of uterus after delivery some time in puerperium, usually w/in hours to days of delivery
- *Incidence:* 1/6,000 deliveries

DIAGNOSIS

History
- Usually unhelpful
- Ask about personal/family Hx of excessive blood loss at surgery, delivery

Physical examination
- Check maternal hemodynamic status
- Exclude other causes of postpartum hemorrhage (uterine atony, lower genital tract laceration, retained products)

Diagnostic tests
- *Laboratory tests:* check CBC, PT/PTT
- *Specific diagnostic tests:* thrombophilia evaluation not useful in acute setting
- *Imaging tests:* not routinely indicated (ultrasound for retained products not generally useful in acute setting)

DIFFERENTIAL DIAGNOSIS
- Puerperal hysterectomy different from cesarean hysterectomy, which refers to removal of uterus w/ nonviable or previable fetus in situ

COMPLICATIONS
- *Maternal complications:* excessive blood loss (2–4 L), shock, blood product transfusion (90%), injury to adjacent organs (bladder 3%, ureter 1%), mortality (0.3%), permanent sterilization
- *Fetal complications:* none (by definition, baby already delivered)

PROGNOSIS
- Emergent puerperal hysterectomy assoc. w/ 4-fold increased risk of complications compared w/ elective procedures
- Judgment of obstetrician in deciding when to proceed w/ puerperal hysterectomy most important determinant of maternal morbidity

MANAGEMENT
General measures
- Highly morbid procedure; should be performed when medical Rx has failed
- *Indications:* excessive hemorrhage (40%), abnormal placentation, severe cervical dysplasia, cervical cancer

Note: permanent sterilization not indication for puerperal hysterectomy

Specific treatment
- General anesthesia, warming blanket, 3-way Foley catheter
- Blood products available
- Consider leaving cervix (subtotal or supracervical hysterectomy), thereby minimizing complications, esp. blood loss; not possible if cervix source of bleeding, such as placenta previa

Side effects & complications
- Although pt will be amenorrheic & sterile, menopausal sx will not develop if ovaries are left

SUBSEQUENT MANAGEMENT
- Follow-up in 1–2 wk; increased risk of postpartum depression

---

PULMONARY EDEMA

BACKGROUND
- Refers to excessive accumulation of fluid in pulmonary interstitial & alveolar spaces
- *Incidence:* 0.05% of low-risk pregnancies but 3% of preeclamptic pregnancies
- Classified as cardiogenic, noncardiogenic

DIAGNOSIS

History
- Worsening dyspnea, orthopnea
- Cough productive of clear frothy sputum
- *Risk factors:* fluid overload, preeclampsia, infection, tocolytic Rx

Physical examination
- Clinical Dx characterized by signs of respiratory compromise (tachypnea, auditory crackles, rales)

Diagnostic tests
- *Laboratory tests:* check O_2 saturation, ABG
- *Specific diagnostic tests:* consider ECG, echocardiogram

■ *Imaging tests:* check CXR; consider spiral CT, V/Q scan, pulmonary arteriography to exclude other Dx

DIFFERENTIAL DIAGNOSIS
■ Pulmonary embolism
■ Pneumonia
■ Cardiomyopathy

COMPLICATIONS
■ *Maternal complications:* respiratory failure, death, preterm delivery
■ *Fetal complications:* stillbirth, prematurity

PROGNOSIS
■ Depends on underlying cause, prompt Dx, & intervention

MANAGEMENT
General measures
■ Goal of Mx: stabilize mother, resolve pulmonary edema, then make decision about delivery
■ Consider pulmonary consult

Specific treatment
■ Confirm Dx
■ Identify cause
■ In acute setting, Rx **LMNOP:**
  ➤ **L**asix (furosemide) 20–40 mg IV push to promote diuresis; repeat 40–60 mg IV in 30–50 min (max 120 mg in 1 h) if poor response; potassium supplementation as needed
  ➤ **M**orphine sulfate 2–5 mg IV to decrease adrenergic vasoconstrictor stimuli to pulmonary vasculature
  ➤ **N**a$^+$ (sodium)/water restriction
  ➤ **O**xygen supplementation (non-rebreather face mask at 8–10 L/min)
  ➤ **P**ositioning (elevation) of head
■ Follow response to Rx (BP, O_2 saturation using pulse oximetry, ECG, fetal heart rate)

- Antibiotics, if needed
- If poor response to initial Mx, consider afterload reduction (calcium channel blockers, hydralazine), inotropic support, invasive hemodynamic monitoring, transfer to ICU, mechanical ventilation

Contraindications
- Use beta-adrenergic antagonists w/ caution in congestive cardiac failure

SUBSEQUENT MANAGEMENT
- Depends on underlying cause, response to Rx

PULMONARY EMBOLISM

BACKGROUND
- Venous thromboembolism (VTE) (deep vein thrombosis [DVT] + pulmonary embolism [PE]) occurs in 0.05–0.3% of pregnancies

DIAGNOSIS

History
- Acute onset shortness of breath, pleuritic chest pain, hemoptysis
- *Risk factors:* pregnancy/puerperium, advanced maternal age, multiparity, surgery, bedrest, obesity, inherited thrombophilia

Physical examination
- Check O_2 saturation, BP, heart rate (tachycardia sensitive but nonspecific sign of PE)
- May be focal consolidation, effusion on pulmonary exam
- Examine for DVT (calf tenderness, asymmetric swelling, Homans' sign)

Diagnostic tests
- *Laboratory tests:* ECG (S1Q3T3 pattern, tachycardia)

- *Specific diagnostic tests:* arterial blood gas, D-dimer, thrombophilia workup not useful for Dx
- *Imaging tests:* V/Q scan ($\pm$ lower extremity noninvasive test), spiral CT may suggest Dx; pulmonary angiography is gold standard

DIFFERENTIAL DIAGNOSIS
- Pulmonary edema
- Preeclampsia
- Pneumonia
- Myocardial infarction
- Pneumothorax

COMPLICATIONS
- *Maternal complications:* respiratory failure, recurrent PE, death
- *Fetal complications:* prematurity, intrauterine growth restriction, stillbirth

PROGNOSIS
- VTE leading obstetric cause of maternal mortality (20–25%)

MANAGEMENT
General measures
- Confirm Dx
- Search for predisposing factors

Specific treatment
- IV unfractionated heparin (UFH): 100–150 U/kg loading dose, then 15–25 U/kg infusion; check PTT in 2–3 h; titrate to 2.0–2.5x control
- Low-molecular-weight heparin (LMWH) not well validated for Rx of PE in pregnancy
- Continue Rx throughout pregnancy & 6–12 wk postpartum
- Antepartum anesthesia consult
- In general, schedule delivery at 39 wk; hold 1–2 doses of UFH; check PTT prior to induction

- Protamine sulfate (1 mg/100 U heparin, maximum 50 mg in 15 min) reverses UFH, but not LMWH
- *Postpartum:* check PT/PTT; restart IV UFH 6–8 h postpartum × 48 h; start warfarin (Coumadin) (10 mg po qhs × 2 doses) postpartum d 1 & titrate to INR (International Normalized Ratio) 1.5–2.0

Side effects & complications of treatment
- Heparin assoc. w/ bleeding, thrombocytopenia, osteoporosis

Contraindications
- Coumadin contraindicated in pregnancy (teratogenic); may breastfeed
- Avoid alternative Rx (fibrinolysis, surgery) in pregnancy

Prevention
- Prophylaxis indicated for history of VTE, prolonged bedrest/immobility; should be continued during pregnancy & for 6–12 wk postpartum
- UFH 5,000 U bid SC in 1st trimester, 7500–10,000 U bid SC in 2nd & 3rd trimesters; LMWH: enoxaparin 40 mg or dalteparin 5,000 U SC qd
- Oral anticoagulation postpartum

Follow-up
- Thrombophilia workup, if indicated

SUBSEQUENT MANAGEMENT
- Prior VTE assoc w/ 5–12% recurrence rate in future pregnancy
- Recurrence rate increased if assoc. w/ inherited thrombophilia

---

PYELONEPHRITIS

BACKGROUND
- Complicates 1–2% of pregnancies, esp. in 2nd & 3rd trimesters

- Most common organism: *Escherichia coli*
- May threaten life of mother, fetus

DIAGNOSIS

History

- Common sx incl. fever, chills, nausea, vomiting, flank pain
- Other sx incl. frequency, dysuria, urgency, suprapubic pain
- *Risk factors:* diabetes, urinary tract anomaly, prior UTI/pyelonephritis, sickle cell trait/disease

Physical examination

- Fever, CVA/suprapubic tenderness

Diagnostic tests

- Urine dip for nitrates, blood, leukocyte esterase
- Urinalysis for pyuria
- Check CBC
- Consider blood cultures to exclude urosepsis
- Urine culture (>=100,000 colony-forming unit/mL of single pathogenic organism in midstream clean-catch urine specimen)
- Imaging studies not indicated

DIFFERENTIAL DIAGNOSIS

- Appendicitis
- Lower lobe pneumonia
- Sepsis
- Acute cystitis

COMPLICATIONS

- *Maternal complications:* urosepsis (10–15%) leading to septic shock (1–3%), ARDS (2–8%), anemia (25–50%), transient renal dysfunction (25%), preterm labor
- *Fetal complications:* preterm birth, low birthweight

PROGNOSIS

- No change in pregnancy outcome w/ adequate Rx

MANAGEMENT

General measures

- Inpatient Rx (outpatient Rx not recommended in pregnancy)
- Aggressive IV hydration
- Antipyretic Rx, analgesia as needed
- Consider serial CBC

Specific treatment

- Appropriate antibiotic Rx incl. (1) ampicillin 2 g q6h + gentamicin 1.5 mg/kg q8h IV; (2) cefazolin 1 g q8h IV; (3) ceftriaxone 12 g q24h IV/IM; (4) mezlocillin 1–3 g IV q6h; (5) piperacillin 4 g IV q8h
- Continue antibiotics until afebrile x 24–48 h
- Adjust Rx according to culture results, if indicated

Prevention

- Urinalysis/culture for asymptomatic bacteriuria at 1st prenatal visit; repeat urinalysis at 16–18 wk
- Screening prevents 80% of pyelonephritis in pregnancy

SUBSEQUENT MANAGEMENT

- Repeat urine culture in 10 d after completion of Rx ("test of cure")
- If Rx unsuccessful, consider noncompliance, failed Rx (poor antibiotic selection, resistance)
- Antibiotic suppression for entire pregnancy (nitrofurantoin 50–100 mg po qhs)

RENAL DISEASE

BACKGROUND

- Decreased glomerular filtration rate leading to urea & water retention, electrolyte & acid-base abnormalities
- *Classification:*

1. Acute: prerenal (hypoperfusion), intrarenal (intrinsic parenchymal damage), postrenal (obstructive uropathy)
2. Chronic: due to diabetes (30%), hypertension (25%), glomerulonephritis (20%), polycystic kidney disease (4%)

DIAGNOSIS

History
- Sx absent or nonspecific (malaise, weakness, tiredness, edema)
- Ask about diabetes, chronic renal disease, urinary infections

Physical examination
- Check BP, urine output

Diagnostic tests
- *Laboratory tests:* check serum blood urea nitrogen (BUN), creatinine (Cr), electrolytes; urinalysis (24-h volume, Cr clearance, proteinuria, infection, electrolytes)
- *Specific diagnostic tests:* check BUN:Cr ratio (>1:20 suggests prerenal), fractional excretion of sodium (FENa = [urinary sodium/Cr] / [serum sodium/Cr] x 100%)
- *Imaging studies:* renal ultrasound

DIFFERENTIAL DIAGNOSIS
- Primary renovascular disease
- Preeclampsia
- Hemolytic uremic syndrome

COMPLICATIONS
- *Maternal complications:* infertility, preeclampsia (esp. Cr >=2.0 mg/dL), nephrotic syndrome (proteinuria >=3.5 g/d leading to hypoalbuminemia, edema, hyperlipidemia), abruption, anemia, preterm birth
- *Fetal complications:* intrauterine growth restriction, intrauterine fetal demise, prematurity

PROGNOSIS
- Acute renal failure in preeclampsia: 40–50% dialysis, 10% maternal mortality, resolves after delivery (except if bilateral cortical necrosis)
- Chronic renal disease: depends on baseline renal function, hypertension (degree of proteinuria does not correlate w/ pregnancy outcome)
- Pregnancy outcome in chronic renal disease:
  - ➤ Mild (serum Cr <1.4 mg/dL): 20% complications, 95% viable birth, <5% long-term sequelae
  - ➤ Moderate (Cr 1.4–2.5): 40% complications, 90% viable, 25% sequelae
  - ➤ Severe (Cr >2.5): 85% complications, 50% viable, 55% sequelae (primarily due to prematurity)

MANAGEMENT

General measures
- Exclude reversible cause (dehydration, obstructive uropathy)
- Renal consult

Specific treatment
- Supportive Rx: BP control, correct fluid & electrolyte imbalance, maintain nutrition
- Correct anemia
- Chronic renal disease: continue immunosuppression (cyclosporine, azathioprine, prednisone)
- If dialysis required, hemodialysis preferred over peritoneal dialysis in pregnancy

Contraindications
- Avoid renal biopsy in pregnancy (bleeding)

SUBSEQUENT MANAGEMENT
- In end-stage renal disease, renal transplantation offers best chance of successful pregnancy (esp. if stable renal function & no hypertension posttransplant)

RETAINED PLACENTA

BACKGROUND
- Defined as failure of placenta to deliver w/in 30 min of delivery of fetus
- Often assoc. w/ excessive blood loss due to uterine atony

DIAGNOSIS

History
- Rarely helpful
- *Risk factors:* prior uterine surgery, history of retained placenta, intrauterine synechiae (Asherman syndrome), abnormal placentation

Physical examination
- *Clinical* Dx made once placenta has failed to deliver w/in 30 min

Diagnostic tests
- *Laboratory tests:* check baseline HCT, coagulation tests
- *Specific diagnostic tests:* unexplained increase in maternal serum alpha-fetoprotein or antenatal ultrasound may suggest abnormal placentation
- *Imaging tests:* no place for ultrasound for Dx in acute setting

DIFFERENTIAL DIAGNOSIS
- Retained placental fragments (eg, retained cotyledon, succenturiate lobe)
- Abnormal placentation (placenta accreta, percreta, increta)
- Multiple pregnancy

COMPLICATIONS
- *Maternal complications:* excessive blood loss, blood transfusion, pain, uterine inversion
- *Fetal complications:* none

PROGNOSIS

■ Prognosis good w/ early Dx & prompt & appropriate Mx

MANAGEMENT

General measures

■ 3rd stage of labor (from delivery of fetus to delivery of placenta) lasts on average 6 min; >=30 min in 3–5% of deliveries
■ 3rd stage managed expectantly; signs of placental separation incl. gush of blood, apparent lengthening of umbilical cord, & elevation & contraction of uterine fundus
■ Oxytocin does not hasten placental separation or shorten 3rd stage

Specific treatment

■ Ensure adequate analgesia
■ Manual removal of placenta if >30 min; if excessive bleeding, manual removal may be required earlier
■ Failed, incomplete manual removal may suggest abnormal placentation; consider D&C under ultrasound guidance

Prevention

■ Placental separation can be encouraged by "controlled cord traction" (Brandt-Andrews or Credé maneuver); however, excessive cord traction can lead to avulsion of cord requiring manual extraction of placenta or uterine inversion & shock

SUBSEQUENT MANAGEMENT

■ Subsequent pregnancies at increased risk of retained placenta

---

RUBELLA

BACKGROUND

■ Single-stranded RNA togavirus
■ Respiratory disease transmitted by airborne or direct contact; humans only natural host

- Extremely contagious (attack rate in closed population 90–100%); infectious from 7 d before to 14 d after rash
- Peak incidence in children age 5–9 y; only 6–8% of women of reproductive age nonimmune

DIAGNOSIS

History
- Hx of recent exposure
- No known childhood infection, measles-mumps-rubella (MMR) vaccination

Physical examination
- Incubation period of 14–21 d followed by maculopapular facial rash that spreads to trunk & extremities, fever, posterior auricular/occipital adenopathy, arthritis; may be asymptomatic; pregnancy does not affect clinical manifestations

Diagnostic tests
- Can confirm Dx by viral isolation from nasopharyngeal secretions but takes 4–6 wk & rarely performed
- Dx usually confirmed by serology: anti-rubella IgM (appears rapidly & remains detectable for $>=1$ mo) or 4-fold increase in antirubella IgG over 4–6 wks
- Fetal infection can be confirmed by detection of antirubella IgM or viral culture of fetal blood or by rubella DNA isolation from chorionic villi; but testing does not correlate w/ severity of infection & rarely utilized

DIFFERENTIAL DIAGNOSIS
- Other fetal/neonatal viral or parasitic infections

COMPLICATIONS
- *Maternal complications:* usually mild, self-limiting, flulike illness
- *Fetal complications:* congenital rubella syndrome includes intrauterine growth restriction, eye abnormalities (cataracts,

glaucoma, chorioretinitis, microphthalmia), cardiac defects, neurologic anomalies (mental retardation, microcephaly, encephalitis); sensorineural deafness most common consequence; rare complications incl. thrombotic thrombocytopenic purpura, anemia, hepatosplenomegaly, pneumonitis, myocarditis, jaundice

PROGNOSIS
- Transplacental infection common w/ primary rubella but rare w/ reinfection
- Fetal infection can occur at any gestational age; rate of permanent organ damage 50–90% if infection acquired in 1st trimester, 6% if acquired in 2nd trimester; infection in 3rd trimester can lead to deafness & mental retardation
- Absence of clinical signs at birth does not exclude Dx; manifestations of congenital rubella infection (incl. endocrinopathies, hearing or visual impairment, progressive panencephalitis) may develop 10–20 y later in 70% of cases; as such, offspring of women w/ history of rubella infection in pregnancy should be followed long-term

MANAGEMENT

General measures
- No effective Rx for rubella

Prevention
- Avoid contact w/ infected persons
- Rubella (MMR) vaccine produces seroconversion & long-term immunity from infection in 95% of cases; immunization of all susceptible (nonimmune) adults & children remains cornerstone of prevention
- MMR a live, attenuated vaccine & not recommended for use in pregnancy because of theoretical concern of fetal damage

Side effects & complications of treatment
- Maternal complications of MMR include mild, flulike sx, fever, lymphadenopathy, rash

■ Although MMR vaccine contraindicated in pregnancy and 1
  mo prior to conception, risk of congenital rubella syndrome
  from MMR vaccination negligible

SUBSEQUENT MANAGEMENT
■ Anti-rubella IgG persists for life; reinfection does occur but
  rare

SEIZURE DISORDER

BACKGROUND
■ Most common major neurologic condition in pregnancy
■ Incidence: 0.3–0.6% of pregnancies
■ Classification: primary (idiopathic), secondary (trauma, drug
  withdrawal, tumors, cerebrovascular disease, metabolic dis-
  orders)

DIAGNOSIS
History
■ Ask about prior seizure disorder, medications
■ Note nature, frequency of seizures

Physical examination
■ Check BP, proteinuria (seizure in pregnancy >20 wks is
  eclampsia until proven otherwise)

Diagnostic tests
■ *Laboratory tests:* check anticonvulsant levels q 3–4 wk
■ *Specific diagnostic tests:* consider EEG
■ *Imaging tests:* consider head imaging to exclude intracranial
  lesion for atypical or new-onset seizures

DIFFERENTIAL DIAGNOSIS
■ Eclampsia
■ Altered mental status (delirium, coma)
■ Drug withdrawal
■ Psychiatric disorder

COMPLICATIONS

- *Maternal complications:* infertility, preeclampsia, abruption (if seizure >5 min), preterm delivery, status epilepticus
- *Fetal complications:* intrauterine growth restriction, death; increase in fetal anomalies even off Rx

PROGNOSIS

- Effect of pregnancy on seizure frequency variable (decreased 45%, unchanged 50%, increased 5%)
- Majority of pregnancies uneventful

MANAGEMENT

General measures

- Consider stopping Rx prepregnancy if pt seizure-free >=2 y (25–40% recur)
- Neurology consult
- Control of seizures w/ single agent using lowest effective dose optimal but not always possible
- Folic acid supplementation (4 mg po/d)
- Pharmacokinetics of anticonvulsant drugs change in pregnancy; adjust according to serum levels

Specific treatment

- Genetic counseling (maternal serum alpha-fetoprotein, detailed ultrasound to incl. fetal cardiac and spine evaluation) for anticonvulsant exposure
- *Generalized seizure:* maintain vital functions, control seizure, prevent subsequent seizures; transient fetal bradycardia common; resuscitate in utero before deciding about delivery
- Immediate delivery for eclampsia
- Anticonvulsants compatible w/ breastfeeding

Contraindications

- Use benzodiazepines cautiously in labor (maternal/neonatal depression)

Side effects & complications of treatment
- Teratogenicity of anticonvulsants related to gestational age (greatest risk days 17–30 postconception, days 31–44 from last menstrual period), number, dose, specific drug (valproic acid: neural tube defects 1%; phenytoin: craniofacial/cardiac/limb defects, intrauterine growth restriction in 10–30%; full "fetal hydantoin syndrome" rare; hemorrhagic disease of newborn)

SUBSEQUENT MANAGEMENT
- Maternal epilepsy 4-fold increased risk of seizure disorder in offspring; no increase w/ paternal epilepsy

---

SHOULDER DYSTOCIA

BACKGROUND
- Impaction of anterior shoulder behind pubic symphysis following delivery of head
- Complicates 0.2–2% of all vaginal deliveries

DIAGNOSIS

History
- Most cases of occur in women w/ no risk factors; therefore Hx usually unhelpful
- *Risk factors:* fetal macrosomia, prior shoulder dystocia, prolonged 2nd stage of labor, postterm pregnancy, midcavity operative vaginal delivery, diabetes (incl. gestational diabetes), precipitous labor

Physical examination
- Shoulder dystocia subjective clinical Dx
- Characteristic clinical feature retraction of head after delivery ("turtle" sign)

Diagnostic tests
- None

DIFFERENTIAL DIAGNOSIS

- Inexperienced practitioner may confuse shoulder dystocia w/ inability to apply downward traction to deliver anterior shoulder; breaking or lowering foot of bed or repositioning patient may elucidate this problem

COMPLICATIONS

- *Maternal complications:* postpartum hemorrhage, 3rd/4th degree perineal laceration, traumatic separation of symphysis pubis
- *Fetal complications:* neurologic injury (brachial plexus palsy, ischemic cerebral injury), fractures (humerus, skull, clavicle), perinatal death

PROGNOSIS

- Obstetric emergency associated w/ birth trauma in 20% of cases
- Immediate Dx & intervention can prevent birth trauma in some cases

MANAGEMENT

General measures

- Anticipate & prepare for shoulder dystocia in women w/ risk factors: deliver in lithotomy position w/ foot of bed lowered & experienced colleagues on hand; empty bladder, consider episiotomy, avoid operative vaginal delivery

Specific treatment

- Identify problem immediately
- Note time (effect delivery in 5 min to minimize ischemic cerebral injury)
- Call for help
- Create space (lower foot of bed, empty bladder, consider episiotomy)
- Perform McRoberts maneuver (hyperflexion of thighs w/ suprapubic pressure); successful in 40–80% of cases

- If unsuccessful, attempt a secondary maneuver. All equally effective, & decision re: which to do first should be left to discretion of practitioner. These incl. Woods screw maneuver (progressive rotation of posterior shoulder toward fetal back to increase bisacromial diameter & forcibly dislodge anterior shoulder), Rubin maneuver (lateral pressure to more accessible shoulder to decrease bisacromial diameter), & manual delivery of posterior arm

- If unsuccessful, repeat above maneuvers or attempt salvage maneuver, such as repositioning patient in knee-chest position, deliberate fracture of anterior clavicle (by pulling outward so as to prevent pneumothorax & brachial plexus injury), symphysiotomy (heals poorly, assoc. w/ severe pain aggravated by walking), laparotomy & dislodgement of anterior shoulder from above, or Zavanelli maneuver (involves manual replacement of fetal head back into uterus followed by immediate cesarean delivery); such maneuvers have met w/ variable success

Prevention
- Shoulder dystocia impossible to predict; elective cesarean cannot be recommended for all women w/ identifiable risk factors

SUBSEQUENT MANAGEMENT
- Shoulder dystocia occurs in 5–10% of women w/ history of shoulder dystocia in prior pregnancy
- Counsel regarding elective cesarean delivery for future pregnancies

---

SICKLE CELL HEMOGLOBINOPATHY

BACKGROUND
- Sickle cell hemoglobin (HbS) results from single amino acid substitution (glutamic acid to valine) in beta-hemoglobin

- Homozygous state (HbSS) has 100% sickle hemoglobin, increased gamma-hemoglobin, HCT 20–25%
- Heterozygous state (HbAS) has 35% sickle hemoglobin, normal HCT

DIAGNOSIS

History
- Homozygotes usually Dx before pregnancy; may present w/ painful vasoocclusive crises precipitated by hypoxia, infection
- Heterozygotes have frequent UTIs

Physical examination
- Usually unremarkable
- Rarely abdominal/joint tenderness

Diagnostic tests
- *Laboratory tests:* check CBC, reticulocyte count; consider urine, blood culture
- *Specific diagnostic tests:* hemoglobin electrophoresis, O_2 saturation
- *Imaging tests:* serial fetal ultrasound for growth, consider CXR for acute chest syndrome
- *Screening:* urinalysis q mo

DIFFERENTIAL DIAGNOSIS
- Iron deficiency anemia
- Thalassemia
- Narcotic withdrawal

COMPLICATIONS
- *Maternal complications:* increased maternal mortality, abortion, premature birth; (1) homozygote: cortical necrosis, functional asplenism (increased infection esp. w/ encapsulated organisms), loss of renal medulla (inability to concentrate urine), acute chest syndrome due to pulmonary microemboli

with resultant hypoxemia; (2) heterozygote: increased UTIs, pyelonephritis, renal papillary necrosis

- *Fetal complications:* intrauterine growth restriction, intrauterine fetal demise

PROGNOSIS

- Clinical presentation less severe with HbS-other hemoglobinopathy
- At minimum, fetus is an obligate heterozygote; check HbS status of father

MANAGEMENT

General measures

- Check CBC, urinalysis, & culture (for asymptomatic bacteriuria) q mo
- Crisis Mx: O_2 to keep saturation >95%, IV hydration, pain control (narcotics), exclude infection
- Offer genetic testing if father carrier

Specific treatment

- Supplement with folic acid (4 mg/d), iron (as needed to keep ferritin >80–120 pmol/L)
- Crisis Mx: transfusion as needed to keep HCT >25%; consider exchange transfusion for severe crisis, acute chest syndrome (2 U out for every 4 U in; goal: decrease HbSS to 40%)

Contraindications

- Hydroxyurea contraindicated in pregnancy

Follow-up care

- Perinatology, hematology consult
- No proven benefit to cesarean

SUBSEQUENT MANAGEMENT

- Subsequent pregnancies at similar risk

STERILIZATION

BACKGROUND
- Refers to surgical procedure aimed at permanently blocking or removing part of female or male genital tracts to prevent fertilization
- Most common contraception worldwide (>175 million couples, 90% in developing countries)
- 3:1 ratio of female:male sterilization

DIAGNOSIS
History
- Ask about maternal age, living children, prior surgery

Physical examination
- Confirm normal external genitalia

Diagnostic tests
- Not routinely indicated

DIFFERENTIAL DIAGNOSIS
- Prior infertility, advanced maternal age do not protect against conception; contraceptive options (incl. sterilization) should be discussed

COMPLICATIONS
- *Female sterilization:* mortality (1–2/100,000 in U.S., primarily from anesthetic complications) < for childbirth (6–10/100,000 births); hemorrhage, infection, injury to adjacent structures; failure rate 1–4/1,000 procedures (depends on skill of operator, technique used, pt selection)
- *Male sterilization:* infection, wound hematoma, sperm granulomas (<3%); no proven long-term side effects (increased prostate cancer, decreased libido); failure rate <1%

PROGNOSIS
- Safest method of contraception
- Compared w/ female sterilization, vasectomy safer, less expensive, & equally effective

MANAGEMENT

General measures
- Couples should be aware of safety, efficacy, complications of procedure
- Procedures intended to be permanent

Specific management
- *Female sterilization* (tubal ligation) can be performed at cesarean, postpartum, or by laparoscopy as interval procedure
- *Male sterilization* (vasectomy): outpatient procedure w/ surgical interruption of vas deferens

Side effects & complications of management
- Strongest indicator of future regret: young age, regardless of parity or marital status
- 1/500 women request tubal reanastomosis; success rate low w/ electrocoagulation, higher (60–80%) w/ clips, rings, surgical methods
- <5% of men request vasectomy reversal; success rate <50%

Follow-up care
- Unlike tubal ligation, vasectomy not immediately effective; 3 mo or 20 ejaculations required to deplete vas deferens of viable sperm

SUBSEQUENT MANAGEMENT
- Pregnancy after failed tubal ligation more likely to be ectopic (50%)

SYPHILIS

BACKGROUND

- Indolent systemic disease caused by spirochete *Treponema pallidum*
- Transmitted by sexual contact (30–50% transmission during primary or secondary infection) or vertical transmission
- Incidence 5–7 per 100,000 in U.S.

DIAGNOSIS

History

- History of exposure to syphilis
- *Risk factors:* poor socioeconomic status, IV drug abuse, prostitution, HIV, multiparity

Physical examination

- Depends on stage of disease (not affected by pregnancy):

  a. *Primary syphilis:* characterized by painless genital ulcer (chancre) after 10–90 d incubation period; heals in 2–6 wk w/o Rx

  b. *Secondary syphilis:* disseminated systemic disease (rash, adenopathy, mucocutaneous lesions, condyloma lata, arthritis, hepatitis) that develops 2–6 mo after chancre; resolves in 2–6 wk

  c. *Latent syphilis:* asymptomatic period between secondary & tertiary syphilis (early latent, <1 y; late latent, >1 y)

  d. *Tertiary syphilis:* occurs in 1/3 of untreated patients after 5–20 y; classified as cutaneous (gumma), cardiovascular (aortic aneurysm), or neurosyphilis (tabes dorsalis, Argyll-Robertson pupils, paresis, seizures, dementia)

Diagnostic tests

- *T. pallidum* cannot be cultured in vitro & not visible on light microscopy

- Dx confirmed by direct visualization (dark-field microscopy) or serologic testing
- Nontreponemal antibody tests (rapid plasma reagin [RPR], venereal disease research laboratories [VDRL]) become positive 7–10 d after chancre resolves & are used as screening tools & to follow response to Rx; treponemal antibody tests (microhemagglutination assay – *T. pallidum* [MHA-TP], *T. pallidum* hemagglutination assay [TPHA], fluorescent treponemal antibody absorption test [FTA-ABS]) confirmatory tests that detect *T. pallidum* – specific antibodies that persist for life
- Consider lumbar puncture for late latent & tertiary syphilis, central nervous system involvement, immunosuppression (HIV)

DIFFERENTIAL DIAGNOSIS
- Syphilis can mimic any fetal or neonatal infection

COMPLICATIONS
- *Maternal complications:* depend on stage of disease (above)
- *Fetal complications:* intrauterine growth restriction, intrauterine fetal demise/neonatal death, preterm birth; congenital syphilis (nonimmune hydrops, echogenic foci in liver & bowel, limb deformities, cardiac malformations, microcephaly, skin scarring, chorioretinitis) occurs in 70–100% of fetuses born to women w/ untreated disease, although 2/3 are asymptomatic at birth
- Only 20% of children born to women w/ untreated syphilis normal

PROGNOSIS
- Vertical transmission can occur at any gestational age & any stage of disease but more common w/ primary (50%) & secondary syphilis (50%) compared w/ early latent (40%), late latent (10%), tertiary disease (10%)

- Immediate Rx can decrease congenital syphilis from 70–100% to 1–2%

MANAGEMENT

General measures

- Congenital syphilis can be eliminated by universal serologic screening & Rx in pregnancy

Specific treatment

- Penicillin Rx of choice; regimen depends on stage of infection
- Penicillin-allergic parturients should be Rx w/ penicillin after desensitization; alternative regimens (doxycycline, erythromycin) not recommended in pregnancy
- After Rx, nontreponemal antibody titers should be checked at 1, 3, 6, 12, 24 mo; failure of titers to decrease 4-fold by 6 mo & become nonreactive by 12–24 mo suggests Rx failure or reinfection

Prevention

- Avoid sexual contact w/ infected persons; use barrier contraception
- No vaccine available

Side effects of treatment

- Allergic reaction to penicillin (5–10%)
- Jarisch-Herxheimer reaction (45%): acute febrile reaction w/ rash, headache, hypotension w/in 1–2 h of Rx due to release of LPS from spirochetes; resolves w/in 24–48 h

SUBSEQUENT MANAGEMENT

- Reinfection w/ syphilis can occur

SYSTEMIC LUPUS ERYTHEMATOSUS (SLE)

BACKGROUND

- Incidence in general population 0.1%; increased in reproductive-age women

- SLE flare not more common in pregnancy; 50% of women have flare in pregnancy

DIAGNOSIS

History
- Most Dx made prior to pregnancy
- Sx may incl. arthralgia, photosensitivity, hair loss, pain

Physical examination
- Nonspecific features incl. fever, generalized erythema, hypertension, mucosal ulcers
- Suggestive features incl. malar rash, alopecia, polyarthritis, serositis, myositis, nephritis, mental status changes

Diagnostic tests
- *Laboratory tests:* check Coombs test, CBC (leukopenia/thrombocytopenia), renal function (preexisting renal dysfunction is associated w/ a poor prognosis. Creatinine >1.0 is associated w/ a marked increase in the risk of preterm delivery.)
- *Specific diagnostic tests:* check anti-DNA, antinuclear antibody (ANA), antiphospholipid antibody (anti-Ro/La, anticardiolipin antibody [ACA]) titers; complement panel
- *Imaging studies:* consider maternal echocardiography (for pericardial effusion), head CT (esp. if altered mental status)

DIFFERENTIAL DIAGNOSIS
- Preeclampsia
- Drug-induced lupus-like syndromes (rarely involve kidneys)
- Lupus nephritis flare
- Intrauterine growth restriction

COMPLICATIONS
- *Maternal complications:* abortion, preterm birth (due primarily to preterm premature rupture of membranes), preeclampsia, thromboembolic complications

- *Fetal complications:* intrauterine fetal demise, intrauterine growth restriction, neonatal lupus, complete heart block (in 5–10% of women w/ anti-Ro autoantibodies due to permanent injury to conduction system; may require pacemaker after delivery)

PROGNOSIS
- Proteinuria, ACA assoc. w/ increased risk of intrauterine fetal demise, preterm delivery
- Pregnancy outcome correlates most strongly w/ degree of renal injury

MANAGEMENT
General measures
- Check fetal heart rate each visit (increased risk of complete heart block)
- Serial ultrasound for fetal growth; exclude bradycardia, hydrops

Specific treatment
- Continue maintenance prednisone Rx
- Increase prednisone (to 40–60 mg/d) as needed for lupus flare; high-dose steroids rarely necessary
- Stress-dose steroids (IV hydrocortisone 80 mg q8h) in labor if history of steroid Rx in past 6 mo

Contraindications
- Antimalarial & nonsteroidal antiinflammatory drugs best avoided in pregnancy
- Cytotoxic drugs (methotrexate) absolutely contraindicated

Side effects & complications of treatment
- Chronic steroid Rx assoc. w/ maternal adrenal suppression (may need stress-dose steroids in labor), preterm premature rupture of membranes

Follow-up care
- Increased risk of flare in postpartum interval
- Rheumatology follow-up

SUBSEQUENT MANAGEMENT
- Plan future pregnancies when disease quiescent

TERM PREMATURE RUPTURE OF MEMBRANES (PROM)

BACKGROUND
- Refers to rupture of membranes >37 wk prior to onset of labor
- Occurs in 8% of pregnancies
- If managed expectantly, 50% deliver <=5 h; 95% deliver <=48 h

DIAGNOSIS

History
- Gush or persistent leakage of fluid from vagina
- May be increased uterine activity

Physical examination
- Confirm by speculum exam: vaginal pooling, leakage from cervix w/ Valsalva
- Limit bimanual exams (assoc. w/ increased infection)

Diagnostic tests
- *Laboratory tests*: vaginal pH >7.1 suggests rupture
- *Specific diagnostic tests*: ferning of vaginal fluid on glass slide suggests rupture
- *Imaging tests*: not routinely indicated (but oligohydramnios on ultrasound suggests Dx)

DIFFERENTIAL DIAGNOSIS
- Leakage of urine
- Vaginal infection
- Cervicitis

COMPLICATIONS

■ *Maternal complications*: increased cesarean (due to cord prolapse, nonreassuring fetal testing), chorioamnionitis, postpartum endometritis

■ *Fetal complications*: cord prolapse (esp. w/ malpresentation), neonatal sepsis

➤ Increased risk of neurologic damage if complicated by chorioamnionitis

PROGNOSIS

■ No increased adverse maternal/perinatal outcome if labor ensues in timely fashion

MANAGEMENT

General measures

■ Check fetal presentation

■ Exclude chorioamnionitis (temp >100.4 degrees F, fundal tenderness, maternal &/or fetal tachycardia); WBC generally unhelpful

■ Consider immediate augmentation given the increased risk of chorioamnionitis and the well-documented association w/ term chorioamnionitis and neonatal neurologic damage

Specific treatment

■ Limit digital vaginal exams

■ Rx broad-spectrum IV antibiotics (ampicillin/gentamicin) for chorioamnionitis

■ Intrapartum group B Streptococcus (GBS) chemoprophylaxis for GBS(+) status OR unknown GBS status and presence of one or more risk factors (either temp >100.4 degrees F or PROM >18 h)

Side effects & complications of treatment

■ Prophylactic antepartum antibiotics can mask or delay Dx of chorioamnionitis

Follow-up care
- If chorioamnionitis, Rx IV broad-spectrum antibiotics (including clindamycin) until 24–48 h afebrile

SUBSEQUENT MANAGEMENT
- Prolonged PROM (>18 h) a risk factor for neonatal infection; consider neonatal septic work-up, if indicated

---

THYROID STORM

BACKGROUND
- Medical emergency characterized by extreme hypermetabolic state
- Represents exacerbation of inadequately Rx thyrotoxicosis, usually Graves' disease
- *Incidence:* 1% hyperthyroid patients

DIAGNOSIS

History
- Symptoms: altered mental status (anxiety, restlessness, nervousness, confusion), fatigue, palpitations, heat intolerance, sweating, GI sx (hyperdefecation/diarrhea, nausea, vomiting, abdominal pain)
- Triggered by stressful event: diabetic ketoacidosis/hypoglycemia, surgery, preeclampsia, infection, labor, molar pregnancy, thromboembolic event

Physical examination
- Fever, tachycardia out of proportion to fever (>140 bpm)
- Evidence of hyperthyroidism: warm moist extremities, goiter, hair loss, tremor, exophthalmos

Diagnostic tests
- *Laboratory tests:* may have anemia, increased WBC, hyperglycemia, increased liver function tests

■ *Specific diagnostic tests/imaging:* unhelpful in acute setting; *clinical* Dx

Note: thyroid function tests do not distinguish thyroid storm from uncomplicated thyrotoxicosis

DIFFERENTIAL DIAGNOSIS
■ Anxiety disorders
■ Drug intoxication/withdrawal
■ Pheochromocytoma

COMPLICATIONS
■ *Maternal complications:* arrhythmias (10–25%), cardiac failure (50%), mortality >30%
■ *Fetal complications:* preterm birth, intrauterine growth restriction, stillbirth

PROGNOSIS
■ Prognosis depends on rapid Dx, Rx

MANAGEMENT
General measures
■ Identify & Rx precipitating cause
■ Fetal monitoring, if viable
■ *Supportive care:* Mx in ICU setting, acetaminophen, cooling blanket, fluid & caloric replacement, ECG, O_2

Specific treatment
■ *Decrease synthesis/release of T4/T3:*
  ➣ Propylthiouracil (PTU) 600–800 mg po stat then 150–200 mg po q4–6h (or methimazole suppositories)
  ➣ Iodine Rx 1–2 h after PTU: Lugol's solution 8 drops q6h; sodium iodide 0.5–1 g IV q6h (lithium carbonate if allergic to iodine)
  ➣ Glucocorticoids: dexamethazone 2 mg po/IM q6–8h; IV hydrocortisone 100 mg q8h
  ➣ Plasma exchange

- *Block peripheral action of T4/T3:*
  - ➤ PTU, glucocorticoid (decreases conversion of T4 to T3)
  - ➤ Adrenergic antagonist: propranolol 20–80 mg po q4–6h or
    1–2 mg IV/IM q 5 min for total 6 mg then 1–10 mg q4h
- *Rx complications:* digoxin, diuretics for cardiac failure; phenobarbital for extreme restlessness; propranolol, esmolol, digoxin for arrhythmias

Contraindications
- Radioactive iodine absolutely contraindicated
- Avoid aspirin (increases release of free T4/T3)

SUBSEQUENT MANAGEMENT
- Endocrinology follow-up

TOXOPLASMOSIS

BACKGROUND
- Due to infection w/ intracellular parasite *Toxoplasma gondii*
- >60 million cases/y in U.S.
- Transmitted by direct contact w/ infected materials (animal feces, soil) or ingestion of infected undercooked meats; rarely acquired by blood transfusions or organ transplantation

DIAGNOSIS

History
- Hx of exposure to cat litter or feces common; Hx of exposure to toxoplasmosis often absent
- Incubation period of 5–18 d followed by nonspecific sx (fever, night sweats, myalgias)

Physical examination
- Clinical sx/signs of maternal infection often unhelpful
- Clinical findings may include asymptomatic cervical adenopathy, hepatosplenomegaly

Diagnostic tests

■ Isolation of *T. gondii* in bodily fluids confirms Dx of acute infection but is rarely performed

■ Serologic testing primary method of Dx; Sabin-Feldman serologic test is gold standard but performed in only a few labs in U.S. (Palo Alto, CA); indirect fluorescent antibody, indirect hemagglutination, & ELISA tests used more often but not well standardized & have increased false-positive rates; serial serologic testing therefore recommended at 3-wk intervals & specimens should be saved for repeat testing in recognized reference laboratories

DIFFERENTIAL DIAGNOSIS

■ Other causes of fetal & neonatal sepsis

COMPLICATIONS

■ *Maternal complications:* usually benign, self-limiting disease; infection in immunosuppressed individuals can be life-threatening

■ *Fetal complications:* intrauterine fetal demise/neonatal death, preterm birth, chorioretinitis, hearing loss, intracranial calcifications, microcephaly, metal retardation, seizures, neonatal sepsis

PROGNOSIS

■ Maternal infection in pregnancy (not before pregnancy) assoc. w/ adverse perinatal outcome

■ Risk of vertical transmission & fetal injury inversely related to gestational age at time of infection: highest in 3rd trimester (60%), lowest in 1st trimester (10%); however, earlier in gestation infection acquired, more severe the fetal effects

■ 55–85% of infected neonates asymptomatic at birth, w/ sequelae only becoming apparent later in life

MANAGEMENT

General measures

- Maternal Dx requires high index of suspicion
- Routine screening during pregnancy is not currently recommended in U.S., except for women w/ HIV & other immunosuppressive conditions; in countries w/ high prevalence of toxoplasmosis (France, Austria), routine serologic screening has had favorable impact

Specific treatment

- Spiramycin (only available in U.S. from FDA) may decrease vertical transmission by 60% & should be started immediately
- Serial fetal ultrasonography (looking for features of intrauterine infection incl. ventriculomegaly, intracranial calcifications, intrauterine growth restriction, microcephaly, hepatosplenomegaly, ascites)
- Consider fetal blood sampling after 20 wk for toxoplasmosis IgM
- If fetal infection confirmed, pyrimethamine, sulfonamide, & folinic acid should be added to Rx regimen to increase efficacy against placental & fetal parasites
- Infants w/ toxoplasmosis should continue Rx w/ pyrimethamine & sulfadiazine alternating monthly w/ spiramycin for 1 yr; Rx may decrease intracranial calcifications & improve neurologic function

Prevention

- Avoid contact w/ cat feces (no need to get rid of cat but do not clean litter box; wash hands after playing w/ cat to remove any contamination w/ cat feces)
- Currently no vaccine available

SUBSEQUENT MANAGEMENT

- Anti-toxoplasmosis IgG persists for many years, but does not prevent re-infection

TRICHOMONIASIS

BACKGROUND
- Refers to infection w/ *Trichomonas vaginalis*
- Predominantly (not exclusively) sexually transmitted
- *Incidence:* common, up to 20% of pregnant women

DIAGNOSIS

History
- 20–50% of infections asymptomatic
- Sx may include vaginal pruritus, burning, discharge
- Vulvar irritation
- Occasional dysuria

Physical examination
- Benign abdominal exam
- Speculum exam: foul (fishy) odor, foamy yellow-green discharge, cervical erythema

Diagnostic tests
- *Laboratory tests:* vaginal pH >4.5
- *Specific diagnostic tests:* wet smear (increased leukocytes; identification of motile, flagellated, pear-shaped organisms slightly larger than leukocytes); <70% detected on Pap smear; check cervicovaginal culture if persistent vaginal discharge after Rx)
- *Imaging tests:* not routinely indicated
- *Screening tests:* not routinely indicated

DIFFERENTIAL DIAGNOSIS
- Ruptured membranes
- Candidal vaginosis
- Genital herpes
- *Gonococcus* infection

- Syphilis
- Urinary tract infection

COMPLICATIONS
- *Maternal complications:* increases risk of preterm premature rupture of membranes, preterm delivery
- *Fetal complication:* prematurity

PROGNOSIS
- Unclear if Rx decreases risk of preterm premature rupture of membranes, preterm delivery

MANAGEMENT

General measures
- Screen for concurrent sexually transmitted diseases
- Exclude preterm premature rupture of membranes, if indicated
- Avoid antibiotic Rx in 1st trimester, if possible

Specific Rx
- Metronidazole 2 g po single dose
- If infection persists, metronidazole 375–500 mg po bid × 7 d; if repeated failures, 2 g po daily × 3–5 d & Rx partner
- Alternative Rx includes vaginal metronidazole, clotrimazole

Side effects & complications of treatment
- Theoretical risk of metronidazole teratogenicity in 1st trimester (rats, never confirmed in humans); consider vaginal clotrimazole in 1st trimester

Follow-up care
- Check wet smear test of cure 2–3 wk after Rx
- Consider checking wet smear q trimester, even if asymptomatic

SUBSEQUENT MANAGEMENT
- Check sexually transmitted diseases in future pregnancies
- Consider screening partner for sexually transmitted diseases

TUBERCULOSIS

BACKGROUND
- Infection w/ *Mycobacterium tuberculosis*
- Pregnancy does not affect disease progression

DIAGNOSIS

History
- History of prior TB, exposure
- *Risk factors:* poor socioeconomic status, HIV, recent immigrant

Physical examination
- May be asymptomatic
- Sx include fever, weight loss, night sweats, cough, hemoptysis

Diagnostic tests
- *Laboratory tests:* unhelpful
- *Specific tests:* skin testing (intradermal injection of 5 tuberculin U purified protein derivative [PPD], measure induration 48–72 h later; interpretation depends on risk status, not affected by pregnancy); sputum (for Gram stain, culture), if indicated
- *Imaging:* CXR if PPD (+) (exclude active disease)
- *Screening:* check PPD if high-risk (pregnant, symptomatic, immunocompromised, recent exposure, seroconversion w/in 1–2 y, recent immigrant)

DIFFERENTIAL DIAGNOSIS
- Pneumonia
- Nontuberculous *Mycobacterium*

COMPLICATIONS
- *Maternal complications:* pulmonary TB, meningitis, spinal osteomyelitis (Pott's disease)

- *Fetal complications:* intrauterine growth restriction, intra-uterine fetal demise, nonimmune hydrops, congenital TB

PROGNOSIS
- Vertical transmission can occur at any gestational age
- Congenital TB presents 1–3 wk after delivery as respiratory distress, fever, failure to thrive, lymphadenopathy, hepatosplenomegaly; early Rx decreases mortality from 50% to 1–2%

MANAGEMENT
General measures
- No change in Rx during pregnancy
- Rx compatible w/ breastfeeding

Specific treatment
- *Positive PPD /no active disease:* isoniazid (INH) 300 mg po daily × 6–9 mo; start after 1st trimester (do not start in puerperium because increases hepatotoxicity)
- *Active disease:* INH 300 mg po (+ pyridoxine 50 mg po) + rifampin 600 mg po daily × 9–12 mo; may add ethambutol 2.5 g (15 mg/kg) po daily if drug resistance likely

Prevention
- Isolate pts w/ active disease until noninfectious (2 wk of Rx)
- Follow-up contacts
- Bacille Calmette-Guérin (BCG) vaccine prevents complications, not pulmonary TB; not routinely recommended in U.S.

Side effects & complications of treatment
- Kanamycin, streptomycin (deafness), ethionamide, cycloserine (CNS side effects) contraindicated in pregnancy

SUBSEQUENT MANAGEMENT
- Reactivation of quiescent TB can occur at any time

VAGINAL BIRTH AFTER CESAREAN (VBAC)

BACKGROUND
- In U.S., 30% of cesareans are elective repeat
- VBAC safe alternative to elective repeat cesarean
- Rationale: maternal mortality from cesarean <0.1% but 2- to 11-fold increased compared w/ vaginal; morbidity (infection, hemorrhage, thromboembolism) increased w/ cesarean

DIAGNOSIS

History
- Ask about number/indications for prior cesarean
- Obtain previous operative report

Physical examination
- Check airway

Diagnostic tests
- *Laboratory tests:* check CBC, type & screen
- *Specific diagnostic tests:* clinical/x-ray pelvimetry not useful in predicting VBAC success
- *Imaging tests:* consider checking estimated fetal weight

DIFFERENTIAL DIAGNOSIS
- Discuss & document risks/benefits of VBAC vs. elective repeat cesarean

COMPLICATIONS
- *Maternal complications:* increase in emergent cesarean
- *Uterine dehiscence* (subclinical separation): 2–3%
- *Uterine rupture:* clinical Dx w/ fetal bradycardia (70%), pain (10%), hemodynamic instability (5–10%), bleeding (5%), loss of presenting part (<5%); risk factors include prior incision (<1% low transverse, 1–2% low vertical, 4–8% high vertical), >=2 prior cesareans (4%), prior rupture, dysfunctional labor, prostaglandins, "excessive" oxytocin (unknown scar, epidural,

macrosomia, indication for prior cesarean not associated with rupture)
- *Fetal complications:* ischemic injury, death

PROGNOSIS
- VBAC success rate 65–80%
- VBAC success increased w/ prior vaginal delivery, estimated fetal weight <4 kg, nonrecurrent indication for prior cesarean (breech, previa)

MANAGEMENT
General measures
- If elective repeat cesarean declined, await spontaneous labor
- Avoid induction of labor (esp. w/ prostaglandins)
- Informed consent
- Attending obstetrician immediately available
- Able to perform emergent cesarean, if necessary

Specific treatment
- Continuous intrapartum fetal heart rate monitoring
- Follow labor curve for evidence of labor dystocia
- Use oxytocin w/ caution (consider intrauterine pressure catheter)

Contraindications
- *Absolute:* previa, nonreassuring fetal testing, prior high vertical hysterotomy, transverse lie, prior uterine rupture, breech

SUBSEQUENT MANAGEMENT
- Dictated by VBAC outcome

VARICELLA ZOSTER

BACKGROUND
- Varicella zoster virus (VZV) is a DNA herpesvirus
- Transmission by respiratory droplets or direct contact

- VZV infectious from 48 h prior to rash until vesiculation & crusting are complete in 10–14 d
- Primary VZV infection ("chickenpox") in pregnancy uncommon (0.5 per 1,000 live births)

DIAGNOSIS

History

- History of exposure to VZV (due to highly contagious nature of VZV w/ transmission rate of 70–90%, only 5% of adults do not have protective immunity)
- History of childhood chickenpox

Physical examination

- Dx of primary infection based on Hx of exposure coupled w/ clinical findings (fever, malaise, & pruritic, vesicular rash)
- Severe complications (pneumonitis, encephalitis) can occur, esp. in adults

Diagnostic tests

- Maternal infection confirmed by serologic testing or identification of viral antigen in skin lesions or vesicular fluid
- Confirmation of fetal infection by serologic testing, viral culture, DNA identification in chorionic villi, amniotic fluid, or fetal blood does not predict severity of fetal infection

DIFFERENTIAL DIAGNOSIS

- Painful vesicular rash in one or more dermatomes is characteristic of recurrent VZV infection ("zoster"), which poses no risk to fetus

COMPLICATIONS

- *Maternal complications:* death, pneumonitis, encephalitis
- *Fetal complications:* abortion, intrauterine fetal demise, congenital varicella syndrome (incl. intrauterine growth restriction, nonimmune hydrops, echogenic foci in liver & bowel,

limb deformities/hypoplasia, chorioretinitis, cardiac malformations, skin scarring, microcephaly)

PROGNOSIS

- In children, primary infection usually benign, self-limiting; in adults, severe complications can result (<5% of cases in individuals >20 y but account for 50–60% of varicella-related deaths)
- VZV pneumonitis in pregnancy has maternal mortality of 50% (vs. 10% in nonpregnant women)
- Neonatal VZV assoc. with increased mortality, esp w/ infection 5 d before to 48 h after delivery (because of immaturity of immune system & lack of protective maternal IgG)

MANAGEMENT

General measures

- Consider antibody screening of all pregnant women (even in absence of history of prior infection, >80% of women have circulating anti-VZV IgG)
- If antibody status unknown, check serology following exposure

Specific treatment

- If an exposed pregnant woman is nonimmune, Rx w/ VZV immune globulin (VZIG) w/in 72 h of exposure; if VZIG fails to prevent infection, it does not attenuate in any way risks to mother or fetus
- For primary infection, Rx w/ oral acyclovir (can decrease lesions & duration of sx in mother but does not prevent or decrease fetal infection)
- Rx pneumonitis w/ IV acyclovir
- Follow fetus w/ serial ultrasound

Prevention

- Susceptible (nonimmune) women should avoid contact w/ infected persons

- Susceptible nonpregnant women should be identified & vaccinated
- Vaccine is live attenuated & not approved for use in pregnancy
- Administer VZIG to all infants exposed from 5 d before to 2 d after delivery, although this does not universally prevent neonatal infection

SUBSEQUENT MANAGEMENT
- Anti-VZV IgG persists for life
- If a woman has had chickenpox or VZV vaccine, she is not at risk of recurrent primary infection

VASA PREVIA

BACKGROUND
- Refers to fetal vessels coursing through the membranes (velamentous insertion) overlying the internal os ahead of presenting part of fetus

DIAGNOSIS

History
- Bright-red vaginal bleeding, usually painless
- May be accompanied by decreased fetal movement
- *Risk factors:* preterm premature rupture of membranes, funic (cord) presentation, multiple pregnancy, placental abnormalities (eg, an accessory or succenturiate lobe of placenta, velamentous cord insertion)

Physical examination
- Confirm bright-red vaginal bleeding
- Document fetal well-being

Diagnostic tests
- Ultrasound may confirm funic presentation, fetal compromise

- *Specific diagnostic tests:* Apt test (hemoglobin alkaline denaturation test) involves addition of 2–3 drops of an alkaline solution (sodium or potassium hydroxide) to 1 mL of blood collected from a vaginal pool. If blood is maternal, erythrocytes rupture & mixture turns brown. However, fetal erythrocytes are resistant to rupture & mixture remains red. Certain maternal conditions (hemoglobinopathies) may give false-positive test.

DIFFERENTIAL DIAGNOSIS
- Placenta previa (20% of antepartum hemorrhage)
- Placental abruption (30%)
- Other: early labor, genital tract lesions (cervical polyps, erosion) (50%)

COMPLICATIONS
- *Maternal complications:* rare
- *Fetal complications:* bleeding is fetal in origin; as such, fetal mortality is $>=75\%$ due primarily to fetal exsanguination

PROGNOSIS
- Depends primarily on extent of bleeding, gestational age, & fetal status at Dx

MANAGEMENT
Specific treatment
- Emergent cesarean if fetus viable

Contraindications
- Previable fetus, intrauterine fetal demise contraindications to emergent cesarean

SUBSEQUENT MANAGEMENT
- Vasa previa does not usually recur in subsequent pregnancies

VON WILLEBRAND DISEASE

BACKGROUND

- von Willebrand disease (vWD) refers to congenital deficiency of von Willebrand factor (vWF) leading to decreased platelet endothelial attachment & increased bleeding time
- Classified into types I-IV; type IIb associated w/ thrombocytopenia, worsens in pregnancy; type III more severe, does not respond to medical Mx

DIAGNOSIS

History

- Dx usually made prior to pregnancy
- May give history of menorrhagia, excessive bleeding after surgery or dental procedures

Physical examination

- Usually unremarkable
- May include ecchymoses, petechiae, mucosal hemorrhage

Diagnostic tests

- *Laboratory tests:* check CBC, bleeding time, fibrinogen (PT/PTT usually normal unless severe vWD)
- *Specific diagnostic tests:* vWF level, ristocetin tests
- *Imaging tests:* none indicated
- *Screening tests:* routinely check coagulation profile, bleeding time before surgery or anesthesia

DIFFERENTIAL DIAGNOSIS

- Postpartum hemorrhage
- DIC
- Hepatic disease
- Vitamin K deficiency
- Factor IX deficiency
- Preeclampsia, HELLP (hemolysis, elevated liver enzymes, low platelets) syndrome

- Idiopathic thrombocytopenic purpura
- Thrombotic thrombocytopenic purpura

COMPLICATIONS
- *Maternal complications:* excessive bleeding at delivery or postpartum, complications of regional anesthesia (spinal hematoma)
- *Fetal complications:* rare

PROGNOSIS
- Pregnancy normally causes increased vWF levels & thus decreased risk of antepartum hemorrhage; greatest risk of bleeding in immediate postpartum period or 2–10 d after delivery

MANAGEMENT
General measures
- Check bleeding time, fibrinogen, PT/PTT prior to delivery or procedure
- Antepartum anesthesia consult
- Vaginal delivery preferred over cesarean

Specific treatment
- DDAVP (desmopressin) 0.3 mcg/kg IV infused over 15–30 min; repeat as needed (although efficacy decreases after multiple doses); can be given intranasally
- If no response (type III vWD), give factor VIII (contains vWF)

Contraindications
- DDAVP not indicated in type III vWD (ineffective)

Follow-up care
- Consider hematology referral given potential for postpartum hemorrhage

SUBSEQUENT MANAGEMENT
- Continued follow-up by hematology
- Severity of disease unaffected by parity